D1565840

Pineview

Nurse Marie McNeilly,
Pineview Hospital
and
Missoula's Elderly Poor

Stephen Smith

Pictorial Histories Publishing Co. Inc.

First printing: September 1999

Library of Congress Catalog Card Number: 99-75832

ISBN 1-57510-053-3

About the author

**Journalist Stephen Smith lives, writes and
researches regional history in Missoula, Montana,
his hometown.**

Commissioned by John D. "Jack" Weidenfeller,
FIDELITY REAL ESTATE, Missoula, Montana

Published by
PICTORIAL HISTORIES PUBLISHING CO. INC.
713 South Third Street, Missoula, Montana, 59801

Printed and bound in Canada

For Heather, Lindsey, Michelle and Daryan, great-granddaughters of Marie Moore McNeilly. May Marie's spirit and compassion for others live on through you and generations to come

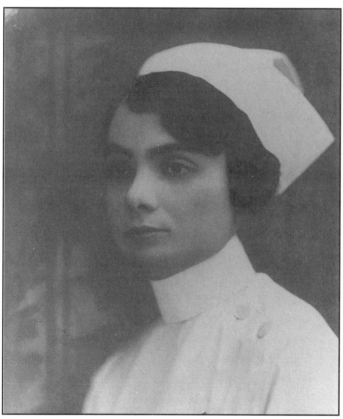

Marie Moore was twenty-one when she graduated from nurse's training and began her long nursing career. (Mary Lou Mackay collection)

Books by Stephen Smith

Contributor to *A Century of Montana Journalism* (1971)
Fly the Biggest Piece Back (1979; reprinted 1982, 1988, 1994)
The OX(ford): Profile of a Legendary Montana Saloon (1983)
The Years and the Wind and the Rain (1984)
Second to None (1986)
H. O. Bell (1991)
Out Among 'Em (1991)
The John R. Daily Co.: Our First Century (1993)
Hear the Hammer (1995)
Pineview (1999)

Contents

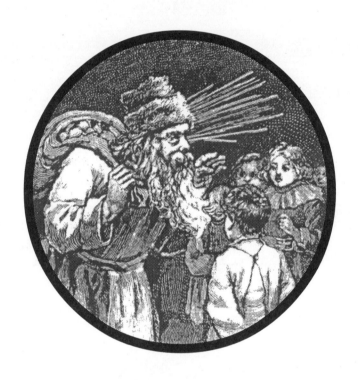

An old man's thoughts about old age

I am in my eighty-fourth year. Old age has not quite enfeebled me or broken me down. The senate-house does not miss my strength, nor the rostra, nor my friends, nor my clients, nor my guests. For I never have agreed to that old and much-praised proverb that advises you to become an old man early if you wish to be an old man long. I, for my part, would rather be an old man for a shorter length of time than be an old man before I was one.

Life's race course is fixed; Nature has only a single path and that path is run but once. To each stage of existence has been allotted its own appropriate quality, so that the weakness of childhood, the impetuosity of youth, the seriousness of middle life, the maturity of old age — each bears some of Nature's fruit, which must be garnered in its own season. Each stage has something that ought to be enjoyed in its own time.

We must make a stand against old age, and its faults must be atoned for by activity. We must fight, as it were, against disease, and in like manner against old age. Regard must be paid to health. Moderate exercises must be adopted; so much meat and drink must be taken that strength may be recruited, not oppressed. Nor, indeed, must the body alone be supported, but the mind and the soul much more, for these also, unless you drop oil on them as on a lamp, are extinguished by old age. Our minds are rendered buoyant by exercise.

As I like a young man in whom there is something of the old, so I like an old man in whom there is something of the young. He who follows this maxim possibly will be an old man in body, but he never will be an old man in mind.

Intelligence, reflection and judgment reside in old men. Age, especially honored old age, has so great authority that this is of more value than all the pleasures of youth.

Old age is the consummation of life, just as of a play. The harvest of old age is the recollection and abundance of blessings previously secured.

To those who have not the means within themselves of a virtuous and happy life, every age is burdensome.

Marcus Tullius Cicero—Circa B.C. 48

Foreword

R eal history, in the minds of many people, is
made at international and national levels by
prominent figures such as kings, queens,
presidents, generals, statesmen and diplomats, captains
of industry, handsome actors, beautiful actresses,
inspired novelists and other writers, profound
philosophers, brilliant scientists and inventors, brave
astronauts and other explorers, gifted artists,
magnificent singers and great athletes.

Regional history made by regional figures
frequently is recognized as significant, too. Local
history, all too often, has been regarded as rather
insignificant, unimportant, sometimes trivial and
usually boring.

In many cases, those who attach no particular
importance to the day-to-day events that eventually
become the history of a village, town, small city or
county are the very residents of those localities. In
other words, everyday people in everyday places tend

to take themselves and those around them for granted. It is the syndrome, if you will, of the comfortable and familiar old shoe. Familiarity, it is said, breeds contempt, so it's little wonder that extraordinary deeds or achievements on the part of ordinary folks in out-of-the-way places sometimes are met with indifference, even mild resentment: *The Wright Brothers? Yep, they run a little bicycle shop right here in Dayton. Folks in these parts think of Orville and Wilbur as a little strange; seems they've been fooling around with some kind of crazy idea for a flying machine!*

Fortunately, the worth and significance of everyday people, as well as the importance and spirit of place, are beginning to take their rightful spot in the historical scheme of things. One needn't be a Napoleon or a Henry Ford, a Charles Lindbergh or a Michael Jordan, to make a noteworthy mark in life. So-called little people count, too; increasingly, as we are learning, they count in a very big way. The history of their sometimes remarkable deeds and accomplishments is well worth recording so that generations yet to come can learn and benefit.

That brings me to our town, Missoula, Montana, and to an extraordinary woman, Marie Moore McNeilly. Marie McNeilly is one of those "little" people, those everyday people, those ordinary people in ordinary places, who, in retrospect, turn out to be giants. Marie McNeilly made a difference, a huge difference, in the life of this community. She never set out to make history, but in her own way she made it. One aim of this book is to recognize her contributions to Missoula and to the human family. Another is to record something of her life for posterity.

Marie made her most important contribution at a place in Missoula called Pineview Hospital, later known as Pineview Nursing Home. *Pineview:* The name suggests natural beauty, which was in abundance since the institution was in a lovely, forested setting north of town. Unfortunately, not everything connected with Pineview and a preceding institution in the same locale was beautiful. The preceding institution was popularly known, even on maps, as the Missoula County Poor Farm. On the poor farm property were buildings known for years as "pest houses." In fairness to Missoula, many communities across early and mid-twentieth-century America had their poor farms for the indigent and their pest houses for those with communicable diseases.

In Missoula's earlier years, there were no facilities in the general hospitals to care for patients with deadly communicable diseases. Instead, people with these diseases — young or old — simply were isolated from the community and sent to a county-owned place, a pest house. Although friends or family members frequently cared for these people until they were well or until they died, the patients or their families were charged for hospital care the same as they would have been in the city's general hospitals.

Replacing the pest houses in about 1909 was the Missoula County Detention Hospital. The detention hospital, like the pest houses, was on county poor farm property. The detention hospital was the facility that came to be known as Pineview Hospital. The entire poor farm complex — including the old pest houses and their successor, the detention hospital, or Pineview Hospital — was sufficiently far from town that a grim motto might have applied to its residents: Out of sight, out of mind.

Jacob Zimmerman, 9, whose parents lived on Missoula's Phillips Street, died in the detention hospital on February 3, 1924. He had been suffering from diphtheria and related complications.

A female faculty member from the state university in Missoula contracted typhoid fever and was sent to the detention hospital for isolation care. No trained nurses were on hand to help her. Windows had no screens and flies were abundant. Walls and floors were filthy. Hospital food was barely edible. The woman's fellow faculty members complained about conditions; only threats of a newspaper investigation and story brought changes. They were minor, at best.

Pineview eventually became a generic term referring to the poor farm/pest house/detention hospital complex. Many longtime Missoula residents came to think of Pineview as a place where the indigent and ill were sent to die. Nothing more, nothing less.

Things changed dramatically when Marie McNeilly arrived on the scene. The transformation was unbelievable, say those who remember. Before she came to administer the facility, nobody wanted to go to Pineview. After she came and assembled a staff that worked wonders, nobody wanted to leave. The story is told of one old man who yelled and cursed when told he was being taken to Pineview. He vowed he wouldn't stay. He was taken to the hospital bodily because there was no other place for him to go. Later, a friend who was visiting him asked whether he still wanted to leave. The old man is said to have replied that the only way he ever would leave Pineview was feet first. He had come to call the place home.

During her years at Pineview, Marie McNeilly received a great deal of help and support from her beloved husband, Emmett "Mac" McNeilly. Marie and "Mac" both gave considerable care to Pineview's patients; it seemed that each individual was a favorite with them. During the McNeilly years, nurses were loyal and staff morale generally was high. There were no 8-to-5 days for anybody working at Pineview during the McNeilly years. If more time was needed to finish a day's work, people stayed without being asked.

Time passed and times changed. Yesterday's sometimes neglected "old folks" are today's active and vital senior citizens. Yesterday's indigents are today's Social Security and pension recipients. Yesterday's poor farms and pest houses are today's modern nursing homes, assisted-living facilities and up-to-date hospitals.

Marie McNeilly, who has left this world, once said there was no end to the stories that could be told about those who lived in the old Pineview hospital and nursing home. Pineview, she pointed out, was home to people from all walks of life. It was home to men and women of all nationalities. It was home to people who had no kin, as well as people who had kin, but were not wanted by them. It was home to people who could not be cared for by their families. It was home to people who had no friends. Pineview, Marie once said, came to be a haven — a warm and comfortable home for many old and helpless people. Pineview, she added, never closed its doors to anybody needing food, shelter and care.

I hope that you enjoy, and learn from, Marie McNeilly's story. I also hope that this book helps demonstrate that local history, in its own way, can be as compelling and significant as history made internationally and nationally. Indeed, so-called ordinary people can be — and frequently are — extraordinary.

John D. "Jack" Weidenfeller

Author's note and acknowledgments

During her working years, Marie McNeilly wrote and published a book titled *The Wonderful Years*. The book dealt with the time that she and her husband spent on Indian reservations in the American West while they were with the United States Indian Service.

After her retirement as a nurse and administrator of Pineview Hospital, Marie wrote the manuscript for a second book. Titled *Do Unto Others*, the manuscript is an account of her years at Pineview, including her sometimes stormy relationship with county commissioners, her friendships with Pineview residents, and her dealings, usually harmonious, with Pineview's staff.

For one reason or another, the Pineview manuscript never was published. One obstacle is that all real people in the manuscript, including Marie, were given fictitious names. Place names were changed, too. Thus, Marie, for instance, became a "Miss Rose." Missoula became "Mission." Pineview became "Mountain View." (Marie used the same technique in *The Wonderful Years*, changing her name from Marie to Peggy.)

As a result of the name changes, the *Do Unto Others* manuscript was confusing. In a way, it ceased to be what it should have been — a true story written in first person with actual names — and took on the feel of fiction.

Marie's motives for changing names is unclear. One can only guess that she intended to shield Pineview's patients from any embarrassment or ridicule they might have experienced. (Marie also changed the names of various county commissioners with whom she had difficult dealings. However, in interviews with this writer for a 1979 newspaper profile, Marie spoke candidly and named names.)

The *Do Unto Others* manuscript likely would have been publishable had an editor been able to remedy the name problem. Doing so was impossible: Marie, the only person who could have "translated" the fictitious names into real people, had been dead for two years when her manuscript was resurrected by her daughter, Mary Lou Mackay.

To write a book about Marie McNeilly, I have used, as a framework, my 1979 *Missoulian* newspaper profile of her. *Missoulian* Publisher Dave Fuselier personally granted me his permission to do so. I'm grateful. The profile has been augmented with additional material.

It seemed a shame to scrap all of Marie's insights into Pineview, so some of her manuscript appears in this book. To be able to use several excerpts, I asked Mary Lou Mackay's permission to change things like "Miss Rose" to "I." Doing so would return Marie's factual story to the realm of non-fiction. Mary Lou agreed. Mission also has been changed back to Missoula, and Mountain View to Pineview.

Some of Marie's observations about Pineview, politicians and patients will be found in a section of this book headlined "In Her Own Words." Several stories, or sketches, of Pineview residents appear in another section headlined "Do Unto Others." Marie wrote those, too, basing them on interviews she had with the residents. That section is preceded by an introductory note written by Marie.

In the middle of the book is a section containing photographs and other illustrations.

About the names of people: O.B. Parsons, Harry Rawn and John Stahl were, indeed, Missoula County commissioners. Amanda "Mandy" McBride, Amanda "Bobbi" West, Della Packer and other Pineview employees named were, indeed, valuable staffers at the hospital. Whether an early-day grouch of a cook at Pineview really was named James is a question not easily answered. Whether Pineview's laundry man was, indeed, named Charlie also is a hard question to answer. Whether Katherine, or Katy, is the real name of a Butte madam who came to Pineview in her declining years also isn't known. Marie used first and last names with her resident profiles; because of the uncertainties surrounding these names, I've chosen, right or wrong, to use only first names.

What is certain is that hundreds of people like those Marie wrote about passed through Pineview during its years of operation. Marie liked people so much, and was so interested in the circumstances of their lives, that I'm sure she took the time to visit with most of Pineview's residents and learn of their good times and bad.

What's more, Marie was a neighbor and friend of mine. During my high-school years in Missoula in the latter half of the 1950s, she encouraged me to come to Pineview and meet some of its colorful residents. Accompanied by her nephew, my longtime friend Richard Geissler, I did just that. I can't remember names from visits that took place forty-some years ago, but I do remember that Pineview, under Marie, was a peaceful, inviting place that was a real home to those who lived there.

I want to thank Mary Lou Mackay for initiating this project. Thanks, also, to Jack and June Weidenfeller, who immediately saw the value of telling this story. Bonnie Flanagan graciously permitted me to hitchhike along on her solid research about Missoula's poor farm. Verna Brown, as always, skillfully waded through my rough copy to type and prepare the manuscript. Kimberly Farmer, as usual, created a splendid cover. Steven Cramer put his many talents to work designing the book.

I hope that you, the reader, will find *Pineview* compelling and thought-provoking — especially as societies and governments around the globe learn more about dealing fairly and compassionately with longer human lifespans and other aspects of aging.

Stephen Smith

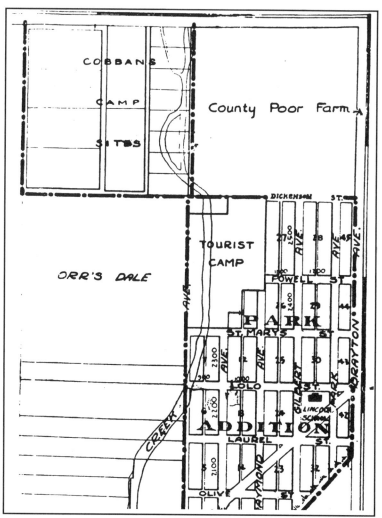

A 1939 map of Missoula, Montana, drawn by former county engineer Charles Dimmick, included the Rattlesnake Valley neighborhood where the forty-acre Missoula County Poor Farm was located. The poor farm property was bordered on the south by Dickenson Street, on the north by what today is known as Mountain View Drive, on the west by Missoula Avenue and on the east by Brayton Avenue (today known as Rattlesnake Drive). Rattlesnake Middle School and Pineview Park, as well as numerous attractive homes, now are on the poor farm land.

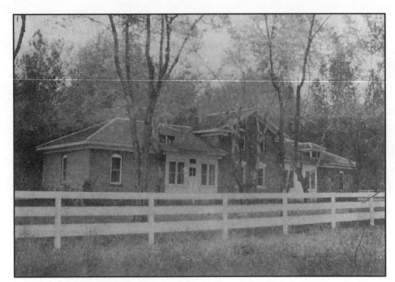

Pineview Hospital, Rattlesnake Valley, Missoula, Montana

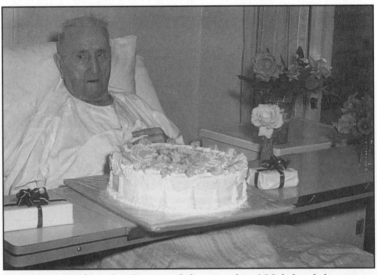

Pineview resident Joe Riner celebrating his 100th birthday at Pineview Hospital. (Kenneth G. Payton photo)

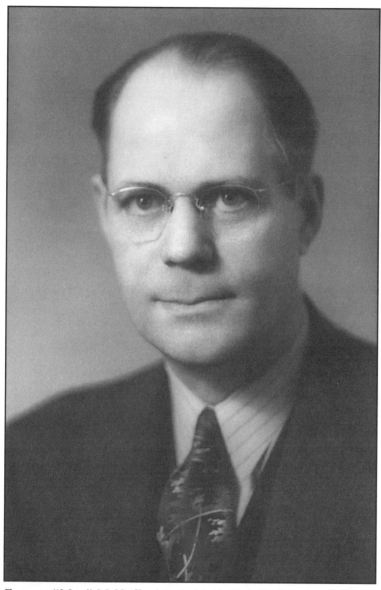

Emmett "Mac" McNeilly, Marie McNeilly's husband and the man who was at her side during her eleven years at Pineview Hospital (Mary Lou Mackay collection)

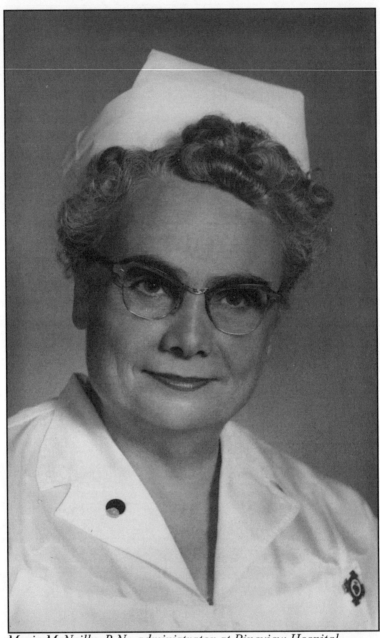

Marie McNeilly, R.N., administrator at Pineview Hospital

1

I was frozen in my tracks when I got my first look inside Pineview Hospital.

— Marie McNeilly

Had she not been stunned by what she saw and smelled, registered nurse Marie McNeilly would have turned and fled from Pineview Hospital.

Instead, she stayed for eleven years. In doing so, she brought comfort, happiness and a measure of peace to the ill and indigent elderly people of a town that, for the most part, had chosen not to care.

The yard surrounding Pineview, an old brick building situated in tall pine trees along scenic Rattlesnake Creek north of Missoula, Montana, was snow-covered on the cold March 1 morning in 1947 that Marie arrived at the hospital. She was supervisor of nurses at Missoula's Thornton Hospital. She had

1

agreed to look at Pineview with an eye toward becoming its administrator. She was to meet County Commissioner O.B. Parsons there; he would show her the institution and describe its problems.

"We started to go into the hospital together," Marie said during a 1979 interview with a newspaper reporter. "Mr. Parsons opened the door to let me in, but he couldn't stand the odor that was coming from patients who had not been taken care of. So, he pushed me in and closed the door and took off for better places. That was my introduction to Pineview."

Marie stared in astonishment down an empty corridor. She fought to control a wave of nausea brought on by the odor of human filth. Then, unescorted, she set out to tour the building.

The first open door she came to led to the employees' dining room. Seated at a table were two middle-aged Indian men. They were having breakfast. Marie gaped at them. Considering the smell inside the hospital, she wondered how they could eat. Marie introduced herself. The only response from the men was a grunt; they continued with their breakfast, never looking up.

In the kitchen was a small, thin man standing in front of a stove. He was stirring a potful of oatmeal mush. His clothes were dirty, his eyes bloodshot. He was toothless. He looked up at Marie, who was dressed in a starched white uniform and cap.

"What in the hell are you doing here all dressed up like that?" the man asked.

Marie tried to explain, but she was speechless.

"Don't just stand there like a dummy," the cook commanded. "Take them trays to the guys in bed and feed 'em. Make 'em eat, too."

Marie picked up a tray. She started down the hallway.

"Come back here and get another tray!" the cook called after her. "You can carry two of them."

Marie picked up another tray and started down the corridor again. She entered a ward containing six old men, all of them bedridden and unshaven. She was greeting the men when the cook entered with two more trays. He glared at Marie. "The county isn't paying you to visit with them guys," he said. "Come on and get the rest of the trays."

Marie continued to carry trays to the hospital's thirty-two patients.

"The thing that impressed me was the surprise on their faces when I walked into the wards," she said. "They all commented at having a new employee who gave them a smile and said good morning. They seemed surprised that anyone would give them the time of day."

What Marie had seen in her first moments at Pineview was nothing compared to what she was to see for the remainder of the day as she evaluated the situation.

"There just didn't seem to be any place to start," she said. "The filth was just unbelievable. The patients hadn't been cleaned and the beds were wet — they had been for a long time. I thought, here is a situation that is far beyond my capability of doing anything about. I'd look at one face and I'd look at another; they were crying out for help. I knew then that I was there to do a job, and the quicker I got started the better things would be."

Marie went to the linen closet; there were no clean sheets. She went to the laundry room and found only dirty sheets: "There wasn't a clean sheet in the house. I called downtown to the county commissioners and told them what I had run into. I told them that the man who did the laundry was over in his room in the basement of the nurse's home and had been there for several days — dead drunk. Mr. Parsons gave me permission to go down to Penney's and get some sheets. I went down and bought every sheet they had, then I went back to the hospital and started with the worst patients."

Alone in the hospital except for the cook, Marie began bathing patients and changing their beds: "I found bed sores on patients' shoulders, up and down their backs and on their buttocks. They were deep, deep sores and the flies had been in them. And there were live maggots. Some of the patients' heels were to the bone with bed sores. Some of the patients were paralyzed and unable to take care of themselves. I didn't get them all bathed the first day, just a small part of them. But they knew that tomorrow was another day and that their bath was coming. It took days and days to get them halfway comfortable."

Days turned into weeks, weeks into months and months into years as Marie, having hired some nurses from Missoula's hospitals, worked to remedy problems that had accumulated at Pineview since the day it had begun to be thought of as the successor to Missoula County's "pest houses." In earlier times, facilities going by this callous, ugly name were used as virtual warehouses for people with communicable diseases.

Marie eventually persuaded the commissioners to match local hospital wages in hiring personnel for Pineview. As for herself, she had been hired for $235 a month to be Pineview's administrator. It was a job she soon discovered required her to be on call twenty-four hours a day, seven days a week.

Changes came slowly, but steadily. Pineview's truculent cook left soon after Marie's arrival; he was replaced by a woman named Amanda "Mandy" McBride. She, in turn, hired a relief cook and a dishwasher. Later, a Missoula beautician named Amanda "Bobbi" West joined the staff. The resourceful and energetic Mrs. West had expressed an interest in learning to be a nurse's aide; over the years she would become what Marie called her "right-hand man" at Pineview. Some other Pineview employees who would be remembered for their service to the hospital include night nurse Della Packer; registered nurses Myrtice Richards and June Woodward; licensed practical nurse Louise Salter; Louise's daughter, nurse aide Charlene Salter (now an R.N.); cook Pheroda Burnett; janitor Frank Rathburn and handyman Bud Woodward.

Perhaps the most frustrating part of Marie's job at Pineview Hospital was dealing with an apathetic public, not to mention an occasional apathetic county commissioner.

"There was apathy at first," Marie said, "but when people learned that there had been a member of the university faculty who had typhoid fever and who was sent to Pineview for isolation care, they began to change. It took a long time, though. The *Missoulian* newspaper had made some threats about smearing the front pages with stories about Pineview's conditions. Then, after I got up there, everyone in town seemed to think, 'Well, there's a nurse there now, everything will be all right.' I got very discouraged and thought, 'I don't think people care.' But when I got a letter from the business and professional women's organization thanking the staff and me for cleaning up the hospital and making the patients comfortable and happy, I took a new lease on life."

The commissioners, Marie said, "weren't very happy with me. I had to have a showdown with them every now and then."

Marie said that while two commissioners — Harry Rawn and John Stahl — were "very good about wanting the patients taken care of, a third, O.B. Parsons, was very conscious about spending a dollar that didn't have to be spent."

The subject of money for Pineview would come up frequently during Marie's years at the institution.

2

Those pest houses weren't pretty. No matter what kind of disease you had, you were mixed in with everybody else. Most of the people who went to the pest houses didn't survive to tell the story.

— Eloise Jackman Pape, who grew up in the Rattlesnake Valley

Money — specifically, public money from Missoula County taxpayers —was a crucial factor affecting the poor farm/pest house/ Pineview operation from the beginning.

A Missoula woman, Bonnie Flanagan, documented that fact in the mid-1980s. Bonnie, who resides in the Rattlesnake Valley with her husband, Larry, was doing research in connection with a Rattlesnake Valley schools history project. Her part of the project dealt with Lincoln School (now the Lincoln School Baptist Church) on Lolo Street. Her inquiries led her to discover that another Lincoln School building, the original, once stood on poor farm property farther up the valley. The more she looked into the original Lincoln schoolhouse, the more fascinated she became with the poor farm, itself.

Bonnie's poor farm research encompassed minutes from county commissioner meetings, as well as visits to the clerk and recorder's office, the University of Montana archives, the UM microfilm department, the city-county library and U.S. Forest Service photo archives in Missoula. She also went through old Missoula city directories and interviewed several Rattlesnake Valley residents. Her research resulted in an unpublished report titled "Missoula County Poor Farm." The report is on file in the Montana Collection at the Missoula library's reference department.

Here, with Bonnie's permission, are excerpts:

*T*he need for a Missoula poor farm was discussed in the late 1800s, when it was realized there should be a place to send . . . indigent people who . . . for some reason were unable to take care of themselves. On March 6, 1888, the Missoula County commissioners discussed a site for a poor farm and on August 1, 1888, forty acres were purchased from Henry C. Hollenbeck for $1,200. That site was the N.E. quarter of the N.W. quarter of Section 14, Township 13, Range 19, in Missoula County, about two and one-fourth miles up the Rattlesnake Valley.

On July 16, 1888, the county clerk advertised for bids to build a twenty-room, brick building for

8

*about twenty residents. A.J. Gibson, a prominent
Missoula architect, designed the building and the firm
of Selander and Gibson constructed it for the sum of
$6,225. By December 5, 1888, the poor farm building
was completed and furnished. A nun, Sister Mary
Louis, was in charge. (The poor farm didn't have its
own doctor. Instead, a doctor from Missoula visited
the farm every two to three weeks.)*

*To obtain admission to the poor farm, a person,
or representative for that person, could fill out a
pauper's application for county aid. If this application
was accepted, the person was admitted to the poor
farm. Some patients stayed for years, others only
days. The patients at the poor farm did some work so
as to make the operation somewhat self-sufficient.
They planted and tended gardens, had a few animals,
helped clean and, in fact, dug graves and buried
patients who died while in the care of the poor farm.
On April 6, 1908, an interesting note appears in the
county commissioner minutes:*

**It is hereby ordered that no
more Chinamen be buried on the
County Poor Farm unless, at the time
of their death, they are in the charges
of the county.**

*In fact, when excavations were made for
Rattlesnake School, Chinese artifacts and a skeleton
were found, so the Chinese cemetery must have been
located in the northeast corner of the poor farm
property. There are said to have been two cemeteries*

9

on the property, but the exact locations could not be determined. **(See Appendix, page 107)**

In September 1897, the county advertised for bids to build a pest house on the poor farm property. It was to be brick, twenty feet by twenty-four feet, with a hall through the building. Plans called for a door and a window for each room, with a transom over each door. The rooms were to be well-ventilated. The contract, amid protests from citizens of the Rattlesnake Valley, was let to J.G. Ambrose and J.B. Truden for the sum of $490. The pest house was to be completed on or before November 20, 1897.

Another pest house was built in the spring of 1899. It was a one-story, brick building with six rooms, iron shutters, a tin roof and a stone foundation. George Dildine constructed this building for $925.

There were said to be other small houses on the property where people with contagious diseases would go to be quarantined. They were taken care of by friends or members of their families. Food and supplies (from the county) were left outside the buildings for the people tending patients to retrieve. After the patient recovered, or died, the building would be scrubbed down and disinfected.

In May 1905, plans were drawn by A.J. Gibson for a thirty-foot-by-thirty-foot addition to the poor farm house. The building was to be constructed of sanded brick, two stories and basement, four rooms on the first and second floor. It appears that bathrooms were added to the structure at this time. This was the last major construction at the poor farm. The years from 1905 to 1936 indicate maintenance activity only

— overhauling the heating plant, delivering wood and coal, and alterations to bathrooms in 1926.

On March 7, 1908, bids were called for the building of a detention hospital on the poor farm property . . . E.S. Newton received the contract to build the hospital for the sum of $6,500. The Missoula County Detention Hospital (later known as Pineview Hospital) was used to take care of patients in the care of the county.

On June 16, 1926, C.J. Forbis designed an extension to the hospital. Builder John Karlberg received the contract in the amount of $6,349. Another addition was made to the hospital in October 1933. That contract was awarded to Charles H. Pew in the amount of $2,695.

From 1903 to 1936, several superintendents ran the poor farm. In order these include F.A. Mix, Lewis Maxwell, Cornelius Maher, Peter Seaton, F.M. Keim, Mrs. L.C. McGuire, M.H. Coultas and Lorena Coultas. Monthly salaries for the superintendents ranged from $125 to $225. In 1918 J.R. Roderick, a cook, received $60.30 a month; Mrs. T.A. Blackmore, another cook, received $10.95.

Lucille Klapwyk was a cook at the poor farm for several years during the Depression. She said the day started at about 6 a.m., with the cooking of a full breakfast, and ended about 8 p.m. after dinner cleanup. Cooks fixed three meals a day for about forty old men (only occasionally was there a woman patient). It was a hard job and lifting all the supplies needed to feed that many people was strenuous.

11

During the Depression, the $40-a-month salary was considered pretty good.

During its fifty-five years of operation, the detention hospital had several administrators. Those listed in the city directory include George Baumgartner, J.B. LaPage, Blanche McCarthy, Yvonne O'Brien, Margaret Peterson and Marie McNeilly. Sometimes the superintendent for the poor farm also was listed as superintendent, or administrator, for the detention hospital. This was the case with Cornelius Maher in 1910 and Peter Seaton in 1911. The hospital administrator's salary in 1933 was $130 a month.

On October 3, 1936, the poor farm building burned to the ground. Residents were transferred to area nursing homes and city hospitals when the county decided not to replace the building. Others were moved to the nearby detention hospital.

T he poor farm, as an operating entity, was permanently out of commission as a result of the 1936 fire. Also defunct, for all intents and purposes, was the infamous pest-house complex on the forty-acre poor farm property. That left the detention hospital, which was evolving into Pineview, and a lot of vacant land. In the late 1940s and into the 50s, Missoula County would lease the land to the Western Montana Dairy Breeders Association, a farmers cooperative formed in 1947. **(See Appendix, page 118)**

Still being operated by the county and still a place of squalid conditions for its aged and indigent inhabitants, Pineview Hospital awaited the touch of a

Marie McNeilly. World War II had ended in 1945 and now it was 1946.

Notice to Bidders.

Sealed bids will be received at the office of the County Clerk of Missoula County, Montana, up to and including January 2, at 10 o'clock a. m., for the burial of all paupers which may die in the said County of Missoula, Montana during the year of 1923. Said burial to include a good substantial coffin and a decent burial, also an iron marker for each grave.

A certified check made payable to the County Treasurer in the amount of 10 per cent of the amount bid shall accompany each and all such bids.

By order of the Board of County Commissioners.   FRED WATSON, Chairman, Board of County Commissioners.

Attest: HAROLD J. JONES, Clerk.
Dated this 15th day of December, 1922.

On December 14, 1922, the Missoula County Board of Commissioners authorized the county clerk to advertise for bids for burial of the poor. On December 15, 1922, this advertisement appeared in the Missoulian *newspaper.*

13

COMMISSIONERS SEEK
PAUPER BURIAL BIDS

Monthly Reports From County Institutions Received.

Who will bury the pauper dead of Missoula county in 1923?

The commissioners of Missoula county want to know and have advertised for the man or men willing to do the work at the lowest figure. Bids will be opened at 2 o'clock in the afternoon of January 1, 1923.

Monthly reports from the county coroner, two justices of the peace, the detention hospital, St. Patrick's hospital and the county farm were passed by the commissioners yesterday afternoon. At present there are 21 inmates at the county farm; 12 quartered at the detention hospital; and seven county patients at the St. Patrick's hospital. During the month of November, 17 were admitted for treatment at St. Patrick's but 10 were discharged as cured during that time.

Four investigations of deaths were made by the coroner's office during the month.

On January 2, 1923, the board of county commissioners accepted the bid of John Forkenbrock for burial of the poor. His bid was $14.50 per body. The only other bid received was that of Charles Marsh, who bid $20 per body. This clipping is from the Missoulian *newspaper.*

14

3

We should hang our heads in shame in this country if we don't maintain high standards of care for our elder citizens.

— Marie McNeilly

From the March day in 1947 that she arrived at Pineview until her retirement in 1958, Marie ran what was to be thought of as a haven for the indigent and old. Her patients came to be a second family, a family to whom she was known as "Mrs. Mac" and "Mother."

For every hardship and problem Marie and her staff overcame at Pineview, there is a memory and a laugh. Marie remembered with fondness an old woman named Katherine, or Katy. Katy had wound up in Missoula after a highly successful career as a Butte madam. She had made a fortune in her calling, but had lost it through poor investments. A stroke put her in Pineview.

"In Pineview, Katy's mind never was quite as it had been before," Marie said. "She thought she was still in one of her houses (of prostitution). She always called me 'dearie,' and one day she said, 'Come here, dearie.' I went over to her and bent down and she asked me, 'You making any money?' I said, 'This is a lot of hard work, Katy — back-breaking work — but the pay is very poor.' I didn't know what she was talking about because, at that time, I didn't know about her background. Then she asked me again, 'You're not making lots of money?' and I told her, 'No, I'm not.' And she said, 'There's something wrong with you, because you have beautiful girls.'"

A week or so later, Katy was sitting on one of Pineview's verandas. She was looking down a hallway toward an old man who was hobbling along with two canes. The old man came to a chair and, after several minutes of painful effort, managed to turn around and settle into it. Katy watched him intently, then she spotted Marie.

"Come here, dearie," she said. Marie went over to Katy and bent down.

"Look," Katy said, pointing to the old man. "It's no wonder you aren't making any money."

(Katy's life story, along with stories about some other Pineview residents, is in a separate section near the back of this book.)

A young Catholic priest came to Pineview to hear confessions one Saturday afternoon. The priest came to the bed of an old man named Murphy. Not

16

realizing that Mr. Murphy had suffered a stroke and was unable to speak, the priest asked him whether he wanted his confession heard. Mr. Murphy's only response was a prolonged groan.

The priest persisted and Mr. Murphy groaned. Soon, from a nearby bed, came the voice of still another old man: "Go ahead, Murph," the other man coaxed. "Go ahead and confess to him that you messed the bed."

The embarrassed priest left the ward. He went to Pineview's main desk, where Marie and "Bobbi" West were working. He told them what had happened.

"Think nothing of it, Father," "Bobbi" West told him. "You're going to be old someday, too."

Several doctors interested in geriatrics were standing in one of Pineview's wards one afternoon discussing how they and other physicians had worked to add ten years to people's lifespans. An old man overhead them and raised up in his bed: "Hell," he said. "Don't be so happy with yourselves. You put the ten years on the wrong end."

Pineview's patients loved Marie and she loved them: "When I'd look at a lot of those old people and talk to them, I felt that they had really started the town of Missoula, which is now the city of Missoula. And they'd done a mighty fine job. They made it a better place for me to live and to enjoy and to raise my daughter. I was very grateful to those people for what they contributed to people who are living today."

Marie McNeilly meant what she said. Pineview's residents knew that she meant it because of how Marie and her staff treated them on a day-to-day basis.

There were times when Marie thought about leaving Pineview. That would have been hard for her, though, because she had become so fond of the patients. Still, it was difficult to do a good job with so many obstacles. For instance, the election of county commissioners who promised things that never materialized; also, a shortage of qualified personnel because of low salaries and what some people considered undesirable work; more and more demands for reports, and no one to help compile them; new and changing regulations from federal, state and county agencies. Finally, the most disheartening obstacle of all — the fact that commissioners came and went.

"There was always a stinker on the board," Marie said. "One who had no sympathy for old and sick folks, one who did not realize that in a few years he might find himself on the census rolls of Pineview."

At one of the times when Marie felt she no longer could tolerate conditions, a brief letter from some local women arrived. It read, in part, "The Missoula County Federation of Women's Clubs wishes to compliment you on the improvement in cleanliness and general appearance of Pineview Hospital since you have been in charge." The letter meant a lot to Marie; now she knew that some other people cared about Pineview and were interested in residents' well-being.

M arie met with the county commissioners in 1952 and recommended a major change in Pineview's operation. She had not completed her discussions with them before the commissioners' chairman suggested formation of a committee to study the matter. The committee included the commissioners, the county attorney, the county auditor, the county clerk and several leading Missoula County businessmen.

The commissioners called a meeting of the group. There, Marie explained how much more efficiently Pineview Hospital could be run if it was leased to a qualified person to operate on a private basis. Doing so, she explained, would eliminate much of the red tape and politics that had become such a problem.

The committee studied Marie's plan. Everybody thought it was a good one. They believed the plan would improve Pineview's efficiency and level of service.

The county attorney began studying the legal procedure for making the change. The commissioners were required by law to advertise in Missoula County newspapers for a contractor/administrator to operate the hospital. A notice for bids appeared once a week for four weeks. The contract was to be awarded to the lowest qualified bidder.

Marie was the only person who submitted a bid. She received a three-year contract on July 1, 1952. She leased the Pineview buildings and grounds from the county, which agreed to pay her six dollars a day per patient for their complete care. She agreed to furnish nursing care, food, drugs, clothing, oxygen, tobacco and personal incidentals. Any income received by the patients, such as Social Security or railroad retirement, was applied to their care. Missoula County paid the difference from the poor fund.

Marie bought supplies from wholesale dealers and in large quantities. She bought drugs directly from national drug outlets and a local wholesale drug company. Thus, she eliminated middlemen who had helped to bloat Pineview's costs.

She upgraded Pineview's staff. She increased salaries to meet those suggested by professional organizations. Employees made some of their own work policies and also some hospital regulations. They felt part of the hospital and were happier in their work.

More important than anything else, Marie and her staff treated Pineview patients like members of a big family, not simply as numbers in an institution. On a day in which an old man at Pineview was celebrating his hundredth birthday, he was asked to make a wish. He replied, "I never want to leave these folks who have taken care of me for so long. They have been good to me and I love each one of them. Now for my wish: I wish to be right here next year when I'll be a hundred and one. Then I'll make my wish again for a hundred and two, and on and on." The old man lived to celebrate his 102nd birthday and renewed his wish to live to celebrate his 103rd. But on December 30, 1956, he was called to what Marie McNeilly termed a "better home."

4

Marie McNeilly was a good nurse, a hard-working nurse. She did a lot for those people at Pineview and she did a lot for this town.

—Lucille Braach, a friend

Marie came to regard Pineview as the greatest challenge of a nursing career that had started in the late 1920s after her graduation from nurse's training at St. Louis Mullanphy Hospital in Missouri.

Born in Flat River, Missouri, on December 14, 1905, Marie Thelma Moore was one of nine children — five girls and four boys. Her father moved the family to Farmington, Missouri, when Marie was a year old.

On graduating from high school, Marie attended Washington University in St. Louis for a year. When her aunt, a grade-school teacher, was injured in a fall, Marie substituted for her for two terms. But she had things other than teaching on her mind: "I always wanted to be a nurse; it was a lifelong ambition."

After graduating from nurse's training in 1927, Marie became a private-duty nurse in St. Louis. But she longed for adventure. To find it, she joined the United States Indian Service. Her first post was the Owyhee Agency on the Western Shoshone Reservation in remote northern Nevada.

"I went as a teacher and nurse," she said. "But the Indians taught me more than I ever taught them."

Young Marie Moore found more adventure than she had bargained for. Her work involved everything from minor surgeries to delivering babies.

"We had no doctors," she said. "We were over a hundred miles from town (Elko, Nevada). We had Model T cars that ran in the summer, but in the winter we made calls on horseback and by sled."

The reservation's superintendent was Illinois-born Emmett E. "Mac" McNeilly, a kind, soft-spoken man whom Marie met the day after her arrival. Marie was to become "Mac" McNeilly's wife in 1933, but in the interim there was more adventure.

Marie left Nevada on a leave of absence to take a course in anesthesia at The Lakeside Hospital in Cleveland, Ohio. Afterward, she returned to Nevada and her job with the Indian Service. Still, she was restless: "I wanted to see California, so I registered as a private-duty nurse. The call I got was from the Barrymore family in Beverly Hills, California."

Actor Lionel Barrymore, who had been making movies despite his crippling arthritis, now needed constant care. Marie Moore moved into the posh Barrymore residence. For the next year and a half she accumulated enough anecdotes about Lionel, John and Ethel Barrymore to include a chapter about them in the book she later wrote, *The Wonderful Years* (dealing with her years in the Indian Service).

"Lionel was a lovely man," Marie said. "He was a real humanitarian."

Marie remembered vividly the night she and Ethel Barrymore sat cross-legged on the floor of Lionel Barrymore's bathroom. They were eating a sumptuous meal from the private cache of food that the actor kept hidden from his wife, Irene. Irene, it seems, was a fanatic about her own figure and everybody else's.

Emmett McNeilly repeatedly asked Marie to return to Nevada and her job with the Indian Service. Finally, she agreed. In 1931, she left her job with the Barrymores.

"I went back to my Indians," she said. "I just loved those people."

She also realized that she loved "Mac" McNeilly. The McNeillys' daughter, Mary Lou, was born in Elko in 1934. Then, early in 1938, "Mac" McNeilly received word that he was being transferred to Montana's Rocky Boy Reservation. When he told his wife, she asked him how long they had before they had to leave.

"There's no hurry," her husband replied. "Just so you're ready to leave by 5 o'clock tonight."

The McNeillys remained on the Rocky Boy Reservation until 1941, when they again were transferred, this time to the Crow Creek Reservation south of Pierre, South Dakota.

They had selected Missoula, Montana; Medford, Oregon, and Colorado Springs, Colorado, as possible retirement homes. When "Mac" McNeilly retired from the Indian Service in the mid-1940s, the couple chose Missoula. Their first home was in the city's rural Orchard Homes area. Later, they moved to Evans Avenue in Missoula's university district.

Soon after arriving in Missoula, Marie became director of nurses at Thornton Hospital, which later became Memorial Hospital and then Missoula Community Hospital. She was employed there when the administrator's job came open at Pineview.

"In all my time with the Indians, I never came across anything like Pineview," Marie said. "I went there sight unseen."

In July 1957, Bonnie Flanagan wrote, Missoula School District One bought five more acres of poor farm land to add to an acre bought in 1902. The district built Rattlesnake School on the site.

In the early 1960s, Missoula County contracted with Missoula Abstract Co. to plat an area for houses called Pineview Homes Addition. Plans for subdividing more poor farm land moved ahead. In August 1960, the county decided to sell forty-two lots, each with an appraised value of $2,500. Missoula

24

auctioneer Howard Raser sold the first five lots at public auction on September 6, 1960.

In August 1962 came a resolution to change the name of Pineview Hospital to Pineview Nursing Home. The home remained in operation until April 1963, when Missoula County transferred patients to area nursing homes. An auction of the inventory in the building on June 28, 1963, raised $4,822.

During the next few years, Bonnie Flanagan noted, there was much discussion about what to do with the old Pineview building and land. The possibility of selling the building so it could be remodeled into a four-plex was discussed, but decided against. Missoula's Chou family, and later the Chin family, stayed, rent free, as caretakers from 1967 to 1971. At various times the building was rented to the Human Resource Council, the Boy Scouts, the Montana Institute of Arts (for a painting class) and the YMCA (for a day-camp facility). Roofs were re-shingled, sewer and cesspool installed, and various repairs made, but maintenance and vandalism continued to be a problem. Finally, the county agreed to subdivide the property and sell it along with the other poor farm property. Thus, Pineview Addition 2 was platted in February 1965.

Concern for public safety prompted the county's decision to try to sell the actual Pineview Hospital building and immediate property in 1970. Officials offered the property at public auction on July 23, 1970, but there were no bids. On September 23, 1970, Missoula County hired a contractor to tear down the Pineview building. The basement was to be filled in, with no damage to nearby trees, and demolition to be complete within one-hundred-twenty days.

Pineview was gone by May 1971. The hospital property had been sold in February 1971 to Thomas C. Haggarty.

Today, there are only dim memories of the Missoula County Poor Farm, the wretched pest houses and Pineview Hospital. A pleasant residential street named Pineview Drive runs along the southern perimeter of the Rattlesnake Middle School grounds. Due west of Rattlesnake School is beautiful, peaceful Pineview Park. A labor of love created from a field of dirt, boulders and weeds by many determined volunteers, the park is but a stone's throw from the site of the old hospital/nursing home.

Springtime and summers inevitably bring families to Pineview Park for picnics, tennis, softball and other games. Always there are children, many little children, making the sounds of joy that children make as they whoop, holler, run free and play in the sunshine.

The children do not know, nor should they know, that, someday, time and the unforeseen events of life are sure to overtake them. If they are very young children, young and blissful in their innocence, they do not know that one day, if they live long enough, they will be old, very likely feeble, and no longer able to run free and play.

The children do not know, nor should they know, about pain and illness and hospitals, nursing homes, medications and health insurance.

26

They do not know that sweet Pineview Park, the place of their play, once was part of a grim place called a poor farm. They do not know that the poor farm had a "detention hospital," a facility to which one man, in 1917, was sent because he had "no ambition," and where another man was sent in the same year because he was deemed "lazy."

The children do not know that the poor farm had drab pest houses for sick people. They do not know that some people who went to the pest houses never left—except in coffins.

They do not know that the poor farm once had a place on it called Pineview Hospital, and that this place was transformed from a sad place into a happier place because of some people who cared about others as much as they cared about themselves.

They do not know about human kindness and compassion. Probably they do not know too much about love—whatever love is.

They do not know about the Marie McNeillys of this world.

They will know, given time.

Emmett "Mac" McNeilly, who for years worked with his wife to make Pineview a home rather than a prison, died in 1967. "When Mac died, the bottom fell out of the sea," Marie said in later years. The McNeillys, in retirement, had lived for a time in Mesa, Arizona. There, Marie served a term as a district president of the Arizona Nurses Association.

Marie remained interested in Missoula's health-care scene for many years after returning to the Garden

City from Arizona. Among her contributions, made in memory of her husband, was the financing of a heliport at Missoula Community Hospital on South Avenue West. The hospital board officially named the heliport McNeilly Airport.

A charter member and past president of Missoula's Altrusa Club and a long-time member of the Missoula Business and Professional Women's Club, Marie also received an honorary membership in the Montana State Association of Student Nurses.

Marie's last years were marked by numerous illnesses. She never stopped missing her husband, a fact that brought about occasional wistfulness and a certain restlessness. She moved many times, from apartment to apartment in Missoula; from Missoula to Wyoming; from Wyoming to Missouri; back to Missoula; then again to Wyoming. Through all the troubles that came with old age, she tried her best to remain the spirited, cheerful woman that she always had been.

She was four months short of her 92nd birthday when she died at her daughter's home in Laramie, Wyoming, on August 7, 1997. She's buried in Farmington, Missouri.

Glimpses of Marie McNeilly, Pineview Hospital and the Missoula County Poor Farm

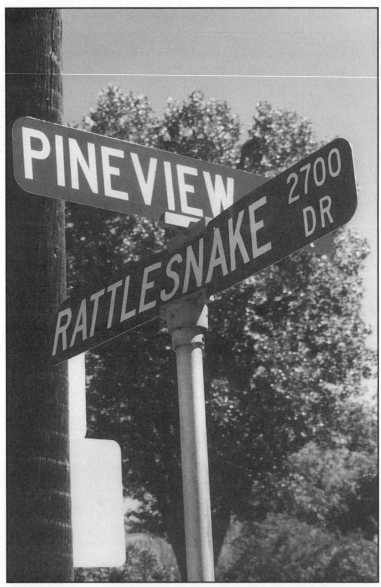

The Pineview neighborhood is remembered in a street sign.

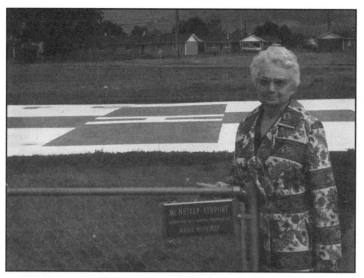

Marie McNeilly knew from her years of living in Missoula that a helicopter pad near a hospital sometimes meant the difference between life and death for an injury victim— particularly somebody hurt in outlying areas. Thus, she financed the first heliport at Missoula Community Hospital. When the heliport was moved to a new site at the hospital, the commemorative plate was not replaced on the new fence surrounding the area. (Mary Lou Mackay collection)

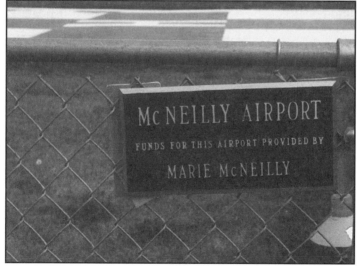

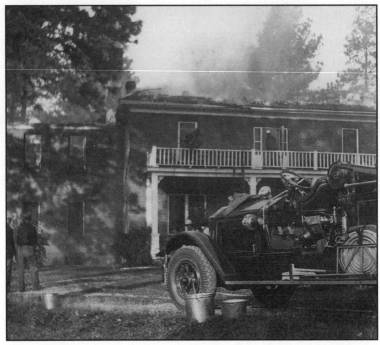

The main house of the Missoula County Poor Farm burned to the ground on October 3, 1936. The county commissioners decided against replacing the aging building. Some residents were transferred to area nursing homes and city hospitals; others were moved to the poor farm detention hospital. (Photo No. 86-0050, K. Ross Toole Archives, The University of Montana, Missoula.)

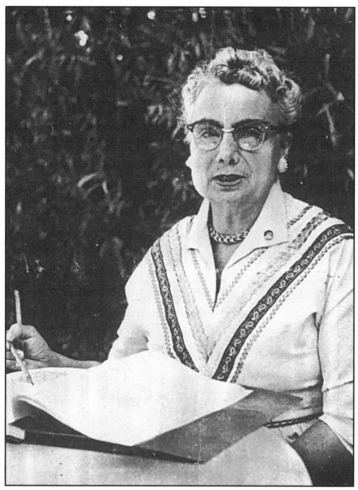

Marie McNeilly enjoyed writing and was an accomplished storyteller—both verbally and in print. This photograph of her was taken in Arizona, where, in retirement, she worked on the manuscript for her book The Wonderful Years. *(Mary Lou Mackay collection)*

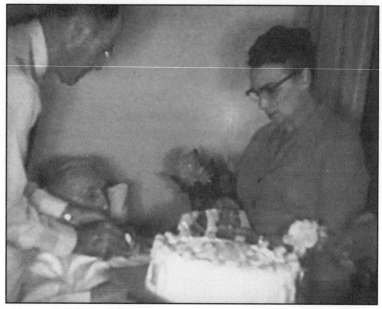

Above, "Mac" McNeilly, left, and Marie McNeilly help Pineview patient Joe Riner celebrate his 100th birthday. Below, patients received ample attention and affection from Pineview nurses. (Taken from McNeilly family movie film)

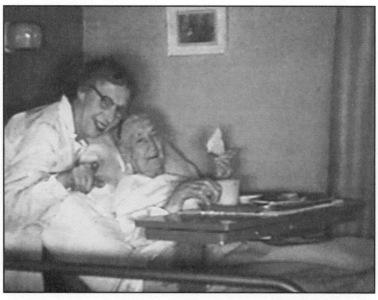

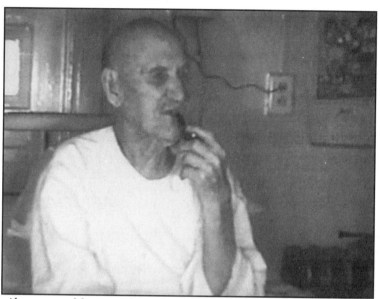

Above, an old man at Pineview enjoys a puff on his pipe. Marie McNeilly and the Pineview staff made every attempt to let their residents have the things they enjoyed. Below, a Pineview nurse checks the temperature and pulse of a patient. (Taken from McNeilly family movie film)

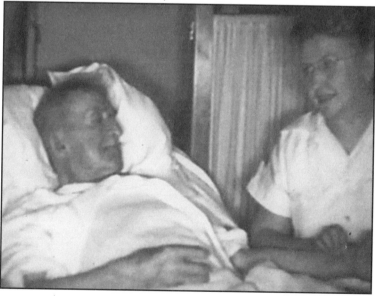

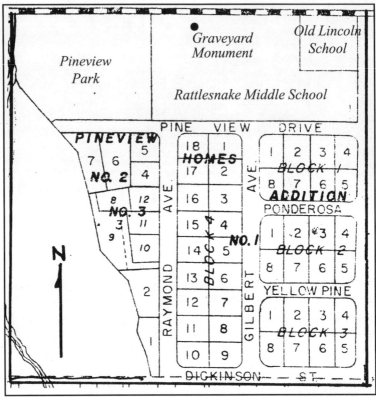

This plat map shows how the forty-acre poor farm property was sub-divided for residential lots. Pineview No. 1 was platted in August 1960. Pineview No. 2 was platted in February 1965. Pineview No. 3 was platted in July 1971. The upper left corner shows the location of today's Pineview Park. The upper right is the location of Rattlesnake Middle School. The small corner in the upper right is where the original Lincoln School stood. Today's Rattlesnake Drive runs along the right side of the map. At the top is today's Mountain View Drive.

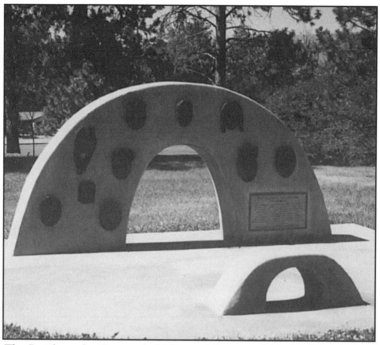

The Rattlesnake Graveyard Memorial, erected by students of Rattlesnake Middle School, is dedicated to "all the people buried on this land." The inscription on the lower right side of the memorial reads: **"People from different cultures lived on 'The Poor Farm' located near here from 1888-1930. After their deaths they were buried, but over the years their grave markers have disappeared. The indentations that cover this land are evidence of the grave sites. Through this memorial we hope you will remember the individual man, woman and child; the poor, the forgotten."**

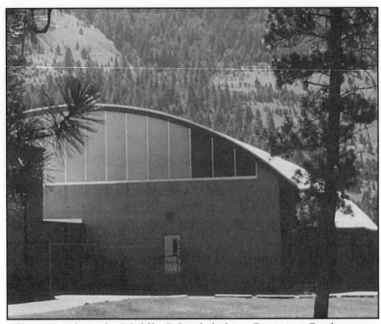

Above: Rattlesnake Middle School; below: Pineview Park

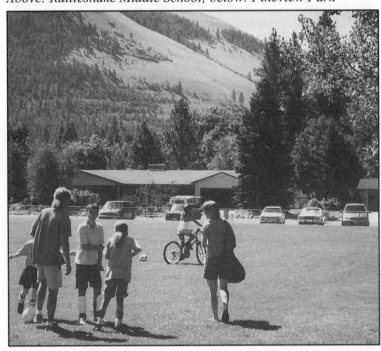

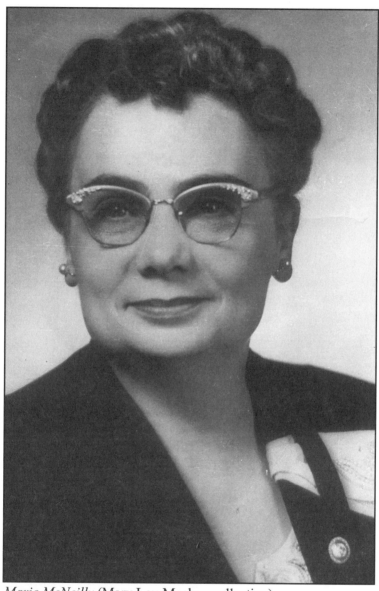

Marie McNeilly (Mary Lou Mackay collection)

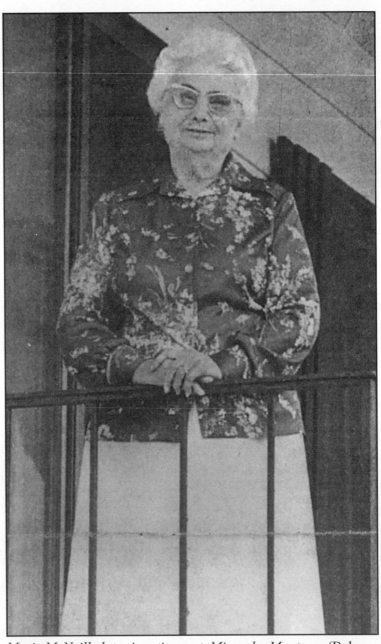

Marie McNeilly later in retirement, Missoula, Montana. (Bob Cushman photo)

In her own words

Excerpts from Marie McNeilly's manuscript,
Do Unto Others

The only part of the crisp March morning that resembled warmth was Mr. Parsons' greeting as he rushed forward to open Pineview's front door for me. His warm welcome came to an abrupt halt as the door opened and the odor from uncared-for, old, helpless patients permeated the fresh outdoor air. It was more than he could endure. He gave me a shove into the hallway and pulled the door shut behind me.

■ I went from ward to ward to see all the patients. There were several who were paralyzed and completely helpless. They were lying in dirty, wet beds that had not been changed for days. I realized that the first chore was to bathe the worst ones first.

41

■ Lunch time came all too soon. There had not been time during the busy morning to think of food. It was precisely 12 o'clock when James, the cook, shouted from the kitchen, "Hey, you, soup's on!" As I rounded the corner on the run, James added, "We only feed twice a day here, but I reckoned you'd be wantin' it done three times a day. Thought I'd do it before you started givin' me orders. I never did like to be told by a woman."

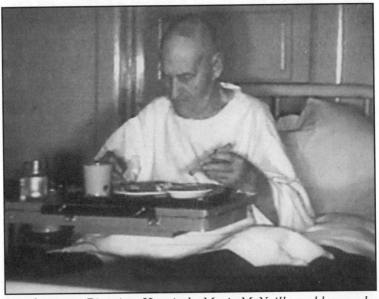

Lunch time at Pineview Hospital: Marie McNeilly and her cooks insisted that meals be tasty, filling and nutritious. (Taken from McNeilly family movie film)

I stared at the trays that were ready to be served to the patients. I was bewildered and ashamed. There were granite bowls, with most of the granite chipped off, filled with corn flakes covered with diluted canned milk. The bowls had been placed in the center of old aluminum trays. Spoons with sharp edges were at the side of each bowl. I thought that being blind, or almost blind, might not be so bad after all.

"Is this all you are sending the patients for lunch, James?" I asked. He stopped his work and replied, "I already told you that this is the county boarding place. You better learn that now; them guys are damn lucky to get this." He hesitated, then added, "And woman, you call me Jim like everybody else does; you don't need to be so damn high-fallutin' around here."

I was in no position to argue, or even answer, so I proceeded to feed my patients with some other food items I found. There were many comments from the old fellows about the noon meal. They seemed to approve of the change. One of them asked, "Is this supper or do we eat again today?" I assured him that there would be another tray before bedtime. I could not help wondering what it would be, but knew there would be something. He added in a whisper, "We go to sleep pretty hungry most of the time." I did not respond to his remark verbally, but I gave his hand a squeeze as I "smiled" my thoughts to him: *As long as I am here, there will be no more going to sleep hungry.* I made the vow to God as I silently left the ward.

■ Jim came to report that Charlie, the laundry man, was much improved (from his hangover), but it would be several days before he would be able to do any laundry. I knew that it was up to me to get the soiled linen ready to send to the laundry in town. Jim volunteered to help. The laundry truck drove up just as the last bundle of linen was tied. I asked the driver if it would be possible to have the linen back by the following evening. He said, "Yes, ma'am, these sheets will be here all clean and we will even have this obnoxious odor removed." I thanked him and he was on his way down the lane with the smelly cargo.

When I started to thank Jim for his help, he said, "Nurse, I ain't a snitch, but maybe I had better tell you that the night woman ain't comin' to work tonight. She packed her things and left for good before you got here this morning." Before I could reply, he was gone. That meant that someone would have to be found to care for the patients from eleven that night until seven the next morning. I could stay until eleven. It would make a hectic, sixteen-hour day for me, but my salvation was knowing that better days were ahead after I had time to get my plan of attack organized.

I returned upstairs to attend to a problem closer at hand — the evening meal. I went to the kitchen to thank Jim again for helping me with the laundry and suggested it was my turn to help him — perhaps in planning his menu for supper. He looked up, startled. Trying to control his lower lip so he would not lose his chewing tobacco, he grumbled, "Woman, I ain't got a menu and I ain't got a plan. The store room is empty except for some eggs, so it's eggs they'll be eatin' for supper. I ain't needin' you now till tray time." I considered myself dismissed and made a quiet exit as I thought of changes that needed to be made as soon as possible.

■ After the patients were fed and the empty trays returned to the kitchen, I ate some scrambled eggs in the employees' dining room. Those eggs did taste good! I made a mental note that this would be the last day for the old, faded oilcloth cover on the table. It had holes in each corner and exposed the worn table.

■ At the end of the first twenty-four hours at Pineview Hospital, I knew that my task of changing existing conditions would be most difficult. I also knew I would be handicapped in raising the standards of the hospital without an ample budget. It was obvious the county commissioners knew nothing of operating a hospital. I was determined that Pineview's elder citizens, old and helpless, were going to receive the best food and nursing care that could be provided. Missoula County was going to get an institution that taxpayers could be proud to have as part of their community.

The second day of my administration brought the "battle of the budget." It was me versus the commissioners. My first request was for a meeting to discuss the situation. The meeting was granted and the three commissioners listened in silence. When I asked a question, they would look at each other as though they understood what was being said. But, in lieu of an answer, all I could hear was a grunt from Mr. Parsons.

After two hours of my explaining Pineview's needs and the urgency of having qualified personnel,

Mr. Parsons rose from his seat to suggest with a polite bow and a forced smile that the commissioners would "take under advisement" all my suggestions. They would inform me of their decision the following week. I didn't move. I knew I had been dismissed, but I refused to accept the dismissal. I was sitting opposite Mr. Parsons at the long table. Mr. Rawn was at his right and Mr. Stahl was on his left. There was silence in the room when I said that I didn't intend to leave their office until I was given permission to hire enough qualified employees to properly care for patients and enough money in the budget to feed them three good meals a day.

Mr. Rawn made a motion to allocate sufficient funds for me to operate the hospital as I saw fit. Mr. Stahl said nothing, but Mr. Parsons made up for his silence by exclaiming, "I am the chairman of this board and my job is to save the taxpayers money!"

It was my move. I stood and looked at each commissioner, with my eyes settling on Mr. Parsons. I said, "Mr. Parsons, I pity you and I hope God will have mercy on all three of you. You have a responsibility to the taxpayers of this county, but I'm sure there is not one taxpayer who would approve of letting these old people go to sleep at night hungry and their beds soiled and wet. I will not be a part of this situation. My resignation will appear in tomorrow morning's *Missoulian* and the reasons will be plainly enumerated."

It was my turn to bow to Mr. Parsons and I did so as I started for the door. Mr. Rawn quickly said, "Please, Mrs. McNeilly, don't leave." He turned to

Mr. Parsons and said, "We should cooperate with her and get Pineview Hospital operating properly. I know the taxpayers want these folks cared for."

I stood in the doorway watching and listening to the three commissioners argue.

Mr. Parsons asked me to sit down. I did. He told me he was sorry for his conduct and said if I would stay at Pineview he would do his best to cooperate. I started talking to no one in particular, but in hopes that they would all take note of what I was saying: "These old people are the founders of our country. Their hardships were many and we are the benefactors of their efforts. They helped make this country a great place for us to live and enjoy. Most of these people are in Pineview through no fault of their own. Any of us might suffer adverse circumstances beyond our control. Let's remember, it's our privilege, not just our duty, to take care of them when they can no longer be self-sufficient.

"We have patients in Pineview from all walks of life. I will name a few: An artist, a painter, a druggist, several farmers and ranchers, several timberjacks. Only one 'did nothing.' The Depression was cruel to them."

I paused and asked, "Do you believe in 'Do unto others as you would have others do unto you?'"

As I stood to leave, I heard Mr. Rawn say, "I made a motion over an hour ago, and I again ask you to allocate sufficient funds to Mrs. McNeilly to operate the hospital as she sees fit." For the first time, Mr. Stahl opened his mouth and uttered a second to Mr.

Rawn's motion. I never did know if Mr. Parsons voted yes or no, but I knew the motion would carry.

■ The third day of March 1947 brought several changes to Pineview. At 6 o'clock that morning a woman named Amanda McBride reported to take charge of the kitchen. She had been recommended as an excellent cook who also had dietitian training. I was in the kitchen when she arrived to make sure that James did not dismiss her before she even had a chance to get started with her work.

Much to my surprise, James did not report for work that morning. He had left during the night. No one except the laundry man was aware of his departure. James was gone and I had not had to ask him to leave.

At 10 o'clock another woman arrived to assume the duties of kitchen helper. She was a middle-aged woman and had been sent by the local employment agency.

That day the noon meal was roast beef, mashed potatoes and gravy, green beans, Jello salad, rolls with butter, ice cream and cookies for dessert, and hot tea.

■ With the exception of the few isolation cases, all the patients who were receiving care at Pineview Hospital were welfare cases. They were unable to pay for hospital or doctor's care. The county welfare department operated on funds provided by federal, state and county taxes. To receive aid from this department, one had to apply to the welfare office. A case worker investigated the financial status of the applicant; the needs of the person asking for assistance were carefully studied.

The county commissioners met with supervisors of the welfare department one afternoon each week. All new applications for assistance were presented to the group for approval or disapproval. Some cases that were "taken under advisement" were, as a rule, just forgotten. One could readily understand why there were so many problems with rules and regulations when there were so many people involved in making the rules and regulations and many more involved with the enforcement of them.

The administrator of Pineview Hospital had the welfare department and the county commissioners to tell her what she could do and could not do. This created a most difficult problem because none of them knew anything about operating a hospital and each one had his own idea as to how it should be done.

A local doctor, Dr. Nelson, rendered medical and surgical care to Pineview residents besides having a private practice. He was hired by the county commissioners and paid a salary from the "poor fund." He also worked according to rules and regulations formulated by federal, state and county governments. He, too, had to please many "bosses," which made his work complicated. Reports were more important than anything else as far as the governmental departments were concerned. It would easily have taken an extra person to write all the required reports if everything the doctor did had been reported.

■ A great change in the status of indigent senior citizens was beginning. In 1948, the first patient receiving Social Security benefits was admitted to Pineview. His check was $54 a month. He turned it over to the hospital to go toward his care. The next month there was a patient admitted who was getting $28 in railroad retirement, plus Social Security of $48 a month. Each month there were more and more patients who were receiving Social Security. Our old people at Pineview were proud to be "paying their way." They had a feeling of paying their way, at least, but the county absorbed the balance of the cost. These people had worked and paid a percentage of their wages into this fund; now they were unable to work and were receiving their own savings in monthly payments. It was a much better situation.

■ The "county poor farm" will soon be a term completely forgotten. As it begins to die, one can see the standard of living among our old people rapidly being elevated. This is one of our country's greatest steps forward.

■ In our hospitals just a few short years ago, one would hear of "the old people's floor" or "the old men's ward" or "the old women's ward." Thanks to progress, one now hears of "the geriatric department."

■ May this country never go back to the county poor farm for old people. It could just as well be you and you and you. Lest we forget, "Do unto others as you want others to do unto you."

50

■ Politics played the major role in the operation of Pineview Hospital. The county commissioners had the authority to make all decisions.

In prior years, Pineview, or the detention hospital, was lumped in with the poor farm. It rendered only custodial care. Knowledge of hospital administration was not important. This situation was now part of the past. The typical Missoula citizen, including the county commissioners, was not aware of rapidly changing methods of caring for the aged.

The common policy for soliciting votes included making promises that were becoming more difficult to fulfill. The first political issue I was confronted with was the buying of groceries for the hospital. Each small grocer in Missoula had been promised a month's business in return for his vote. Mr. Jones this month, Mr. Smith next month, and so on down the line until each had had their turn.

On receiving an itemized grocery bill one day, I telephoned the grocer to complain about the hospital being overcharged on a number of items. He replied, "Listen lady, I only get this business one month out of each year and I make hay while the sun shines." With this blunt, but to-the-point, explanation, he hung up.

Another problem in trying to patronize smaller business establishments was that of supply. If Pineview ordered fresh green beans, only half, or maybe a third, of the order would be filled. When I would call and ask a merchant about the balance of the order, I would be told that they had sent all they had. In a few days, I'd be told, the balance would be sent.

By the time the balance of the required amount for one meal arrived, the first part of the order was not fit for use and there was not a sufficient amount of the second part of the order to serve everyone. This sort of thing happened week after week, making it difficult for Pineview's dietitian to plan meals.

It was in regulations of the state welfare department, because of its contribution to the county welfare fund, that each item of any purchase be itemized on the bill accompanying a claim. Large markets ran the list of groceries through checkout machines and did not itemize each article. They were not eager to do business with Pineview because of the time-consuming red tape involved.

Drugs were to be ordered in the same manner. Each drug store was to have a month's business from Pineview. The cost of operating the hospital was a great deal higher than necessary. It being a county hospital, drugs could have been bought directly from drug companies cheaper than local drug stores could buy them. Instead, drug stores bought from the drug companies, then added their forty percent profit.

I was aware that the cost of Pineview's operation could be significantly reduced if I was permitted to buy all supplies through wholesale dealers. But, under the established method of buying for a county-operated institution, I was unable to operate Pineview in an economical manner. There were too many people who believed they should have their share of the business.

Two electricians were called to do a small job at Pineview. After they left, a hammer belonging to the hospital was missing. I called one of the men and was told, "Yes, I took it. My taxes were high this year, so I figured I paid for that hammer." He did not believe that he had done anything wrong. After I explained to him how difficult it was to get a few needed tools for the hospital, he returned the hammer.

There was no money in the budget for flowers or plants in the hospital yard. I bought plants with my own money and planted them along the edge of the lawn. They grew and were blooming beautifully. One morning a lady from Missoula was seen cutting herself a large bouquet. One of our nurses went out in the yard and told her the flowers belonged to the hospital and weren't cut because patients enjoyed them so much. The woman's answer was, "I'm a taxpayer, have been for years, and taxes are plenty high. These flowers are as much mine as they are yours." She took the flowers, got into her car and drove away.

■ My contract with the county to operate Pineview Hospital expired on August 31, 1955. It had been re-advertised for bid the first of August. After the legal procedure had been followed and the bids to operate Pineview were opened, I was notified that I should continue to operate the hospital for three more years.

Pineview was filled to capacity at all times. Doctors would transfer patients who did not require skilled nursing care to local nursing and rest homes to make space for people who were in Missoula's general hospitals.

The Montana State Board of Health had been working for a number of years on reclassification of hospitals and nursing homes. This was a necessary step in order to elevate and maintain higher standards for all institutions caring for the sick.

Pineview Hospital didn't have space to render all the services required to qualify as a general hospital. It didn't have a surgery, any x-ray department, a maternity department. When patients at Pineview required more services, they were transferred to a general hospital in Missoula. If a patient had major surgery, he was returned to Pineview by ambulance in a few days for post-operative care.

A detailed inspection of the building and services was done by the licensing department of the state board of health. After this inspection, Pineview Hospital was changed to Pineview Nursing Home. At this time the county commissioners received a full report of the inspection by the state board of health. The report included many recommendations for changes in the facilities to qualify for a license to continue operation.

An entire new and modern hospital was badly needed. But this could not be accomplished. Renovation of the facility proved to be much more expensive than the commissioners had anticipated. Seven thousand dollars was the lowest figure they had been quoted. It did not seem practical to put such expensive equipment into an old building.

The major recommendations were "taken under advisement," which meant that nothing was being done.

I left at the end of my contract, which terminated August 31, 1958. I left Pineview running smoothly with well-trained personnel. The nursing care and the food were above average, but the building was old and beyond repair. This was home to those old folks and they loved that old house and the nurses and cooks who took such good care of them.

In 1962 the commissioners arranged with the nursing homes of Missoula to take the patients from Pineview. One by one they were moved to their new homes. The status of the senior citizen in America was changing at a rapid rate. They were all receiving Social Security and no longer were county indigents. Most everyone could pay for his care, or at least pay a portion of his bill. This makes a great difference in the morale of our old folks today.

Many citizens of Missoula protested the closing of Pineview. They did everything they could to save the place. It couldn't be saved; its time had come and gone.

"When I'd look at a lot of those old people and talk to them, I felt that they had really started the town of Missoula, which is now the city of Missoula. And they'd done a mighty fine job. They made it a better place for me to live and to enjoy and to raise my daughter. I was very grateful to those people for what they contributed to people who are living today."

—Marie McNeilly

Do unto others...

*Stories from the wards and hallways of
Pineview Hospital*

(**AUTHOR'S NOTE:** Marie McNeilly wrote
this introduction and the stories that follow. The
stories are based on interviews that Marie conducted
with Pineview residents.)

*S*ome folks "get old" gracefully and try to enjoy
each day of growing older. Then there are those
who fight every step of the way, disliking every
day of the aging process.

*God gave us four seasons: Spring, summer,
autumn and winter. We think of these seasons in terms
of weather and the time of year. Each season is a
stimulus; at the beginning of each we plan, with
increased enthusiasm, our work for that particular
time of year.*

Our lives are similar to the seasons. Spring is birth, youth and reaching for maturity. Summer finds us in the prime of manhood and womanhood with a chosen business or profession or trade enabling us to earn a living for ourselves and our families. These are our years to produce and contribute. Autumn years start around the age of sixty-five. They should be happy years. We cease to worry about daily toil. Our years of toil are over and we can relax, rest and plan to do the things we have dreamed of doing for so many years, but could not do until our summer years were over. We can travel and visit places we always have wanted to see; we can visit our children and grandchildren whenever we wish; we can visit friends we have made during our lives. For many of us there will be an "Indian summer" rich in pleasures and often lasting a long time.

Then we all must prepare for the winter of our years. That is the time in which we may no longer be self-sufficient and perhaps will need somebody to care for us. We may need to go to a home for folks who have reached the winter season, but that should not be a sad time. There are others just like us there. We can only hope that they are well cared for and happy, and that we will be, too.

It may be cold outdoors, it may be snowing, it may be a beautiful winter day, but is there a better time to count our blessings and have communion with God and prepare ourselves for that wonderful day of entering the gates of His kingdom?

Yes, our winter season should be a happy one. These are the days in which we take inventory of our

58

lives on this earth; they are a time for us to be proud of the contributions we have made.

*T*he people who lived at Pineview were people from all walks of life. They came to Pineview to spend the winter of their lives. Most of them accepted old age graciously and tried to be happy.

Many of them helped make this country a better place for us to live and to raise our children. They suffered many hardships in pioneering new territory and building communities with schools, churches, hospitals and businesses to serve their people.

Each and every person who made his or her home at Pineview had a story to tell. Each one had a book to write, but just did not get it written. Our home libraries, our church libraries, our school libraries and our community libraries would be so much richer if ordinary folks like yourselves would just take the time to write that book — a book about your own life and experiences.

I'm sure these stories of every-day people will interest you. Perhaps one of them will remind you of somebody you have known — maybe a relative, a neighbor, a friend or simply an acquaintance. Perhaps one of these stories will help somebody to understand some old person and help to solve a problem, making life a little easier for all. If so, the stories will have served the purpose for which they were written: May they help to remind everybody that there will be a winter season for us all, and may they remind everybody to "Do unto others as you would like others to do unto you" during your winter season.

Katherine (Katy)

Katherine, or Katy, was born in St. Louis, Missouri, on December 14, 1868. She was an only child. Her mother had been a teacher and her father was in the freighting business. He owned several barges that carried freight on the Mississippi River.

The family lived in a cozy, brick bungalow near the river. Men who worked for Katy's father often would stop at the family home and discuss their trips to the river towns. Katy was fascinated with the stories she heard and promised herself that someday she would take a trip on the river — and maybe even far away.

Katy's mother was a very kind, gentle person who loved her daughter. She tried hard to protect the little girl from displays of temper and brutality that Katy's father did not try to control, especially when he was drinking. Her father often would beat Katy's mother, but it was not until Katy was sixteen years of age that he started beating her. His periods of drinking and the tantrums that followed grew closer together and lasted longer as Katy grew older. Her mother's health began to fail.

A young man named Carl Beck worked on a freight boat on the Missouri River. He met Katy at a dance on a large passenger boat and began to show her much attention. She did not care a great deal for him, but found it convenient to go with him because her father approved of the young man. He never had approved of any male friend that Katy or her mother liked.

On Katy's eighteenth birthday, Carl Beck came to spend the evening. Katy's father was on a trip to New Orleans. Katy's mother helped her daughter pack an old straw suitcase she had borrowed from her aunt. She gave Katy all the money she had saved over a long period of time. It amounted to about $105. She had kept nickels, dimes and quarters out of her household money to have when Katy needed it.

Carl's freight boat was scheduled to leave for Fort Benton, Montana, at 5 o'clock the next morning. He asked the captain of the boat if he might take his new wife on this trip. The captain was not in favor of having a woman on his boat, but when Carl gave him $25 he agreed to take her.

They would be many miles up the Missouri River before Katy's father returned from New Orleans. Katy's mother went to the dock to see her daughter off. She knew she was not going to live much longer and she did not want Katy left alone with her father, who was likely to mistreat her. Carl promised that he would be good to Katy and that they would be married as soon as they reached Fort Benton.

Katy's mother kissed her daughter and shook Carl's hand as she pleaded with him never to mistreat Katy as her father had. The mother did not remain to see the boat leave, but slowly walked up the path to her house, which was empty now. She sat for several hours in Katy's chair near the bed. Tears would not come, although the pain in her heart was almost unbearable. She asked God to be merciful as she moved over to Katy's bed. After she had rested, the pain subsided; as she stared at the ceiling she imagined she was with Carl and Katy on the boat steaming up the river. She felt drowsy and it seemed her body was floating through the air. Her heavy eyelids closed and she was at peace.

The old freight boat made many stops to unload part of its cargo and take on more to be delivered farther north. Katy never had felt so free, nor had she ever been so happy. Not because she was with Carl, but because everybody on the boat was kind and considerate of her. She never knew men could be so kind.

Every night an old man named Sam would play his Jew's harp and Katy would dance, first with one crewman, then with another. Carl was very polite and courteous to her, but never tried to kiss her. They apparently occupied the same bed in the corner of a large compartment where everybody slept. The captain thought Katy and Carl were married; he had a curtain made out of an old piece of canvas so they might have some privacy. There was no need for this because Carl did not touch Katy. He very quietly slid beneath the bed and remained there all night. Katy was grateful for this gesture. She began to wonder what Carl had planned after they arrived in Montana, but decided she would enjoy herself and let time take care of the problem.

It took fifteen days to reach Fort Benton and Katy was beginning to tire. She began to realize she would have to make plans for her future. She knew

Carl was a crew member of the freight boat and that in a few days it would be returning to St. Louis for more cargo. That was his work and he liked that life. She knew now that he never intended to marry her and had only helped her to get to this new place to make a life for herself. He had told Katy and her mother about the wonderful opportunities the West held for anybody who was willing to take advantage of them.

Katy never had wanted to marry Carl. She wanted to be free to live her life as she saw fit. The last day of the journey, Carl spent most of his free time telling Katy about the town of Fort Benton. There were several jobs she could find if she wished to remain there.

There was a place called Butte many miles to the south of Fort Benton. A huge deposit of copper had been discovered and mines were being opened. This meant there would be work for her there if she were interested.

Katy said good-bye to the boat crew and there was a handshake with Carl as he wished her good luck with her new life. He carried her suitcase to a buggy that was standing ready to serve anybody who needed transportation to the hotel, which was about ten blocks from the dock. Katy climbed into the seat beside the driver and they were on their way as soon as Carl had given the man fifty cents for her fare.

A job was available in the hotel and Katy found herself employed before she even had unpacked her suitcase. She was to help serve meals, help wash dishes and make beds and tidy up rooms between meal times. There was no running water in the rooms. Katy had to carry water in large pitchers and place the pitchers on the washstands in each room.

She enjoyed her work and made a good employee. People liked Katy and she didn't have time to get lonesome or homesick. Carl had brought her news of her mother's death on his last trip, but did not know what had become of her father. Carl had heard a man say that he moved to New Orleans, but he did not know if this was true. Katy did not care where her father was. She was sad when she learned about her mother. Now she would never want to go back to St. Louis.

Many of the guests at the Fort Benton Hotel were men going to Butte or men from Butte coming to Fort Benton on business. Katy heard so much about the mining town that she decided she would go there as soon as winter was over. The middle of May, she arrived in Butte, with all her worldly possessions. She had saved some money and decided to open a business of her own. An official of the mines explained to her the need of a "house of girls" to serve the men of the community. He told her that this was a legitimate business in the West and a profitable one at that. He also told her he would personally lend her the money to start a first-class place, and this he did. In a few weeks, at the edge of town, was a two-story house ready for business.

On the first floor was a large reception room, elaborately furnished. The floors were covered with blue, velvety carpets. The furniture was upholstered in gold-brocaded velvet. A large chandelier of sparkling

64

cut glass trimmed in gold hung from the center of the ceiling. There was a long fireplace with a beautiful mirror framed in antique gold. Across the hall from the living room was a library containing books and magazines. A long table with many comfortable chairs occupied the center of the room. The girls could spend much of their time in this room reading or playing the Victrola when they were not busy with a customer in their bedrooms.

Katy had a suite of rooms just back of these front rooms. Behind her rooms were the dining room for the girls and the kitchen and pantry. There also was a small bedroom for the cook at the rear of the building.

A carpeted, winding stairway inside the front door led to the second floor, where the girls had bedrooms.

Katy always answered the doorbell to greet her clientele and to collect the fee, which was $3 for one hour or a fraction thereof. She kept two dollars and gave one dollar to the girl who rendered the service. If the customer spent the night, the fee was $15. Katy kept ten and the girl was given five. No one could consider it an all-night visit until after midnight unless previous arrangements were made with the madam and extra remuneration for overtime was paid in advance.

Katy and her girls were not accepted in the social circles of the community, but the "sporting house" was accepted as a necessary and legal business in the mining town. The girls were required by law to report to one of the practicing physicians at two-week intervals for an examination. If there were any symptoms of venereal disease, the girl was not allowed to pursue her work until she had a certificate of clean health. Physicians did an excellent job of keeping disease at a minimum.

Butte flourished for years, as did Katy. There were other houses: The Candy Cane, The Blue Bells, Madge's Silver Dollar, The Copper Bee Hive. Many more came and went, but men liked Madam Katy. She was always a lady — pleasant, honest and polite — and had such a sweet smile for everybody. She was one of the largest contributors to Butte's churches and always was ready to help people in need. She had the reputation of being kinder to her girls than any other madam in the business.

After many years of providing her service, Katy decided to retire and live a normal life. She sold her sporting house and became Miss Katy again. She traveled the world and visited many countries she had read about and had always wanted to see. She loved people and had spent many years wanting to be a woman that a community would accept as one of its respected citizens. Now she could walk up the steps and go through the front door of a church as she had longed to do.

Katy loved Montana and wanted to spend the rest of her life in the state. She had lost her money in some poor investments and now was too old to work. She eventually found a room in a boarding house in Missoula, Montana, and tried to find part-time work to buy her food.

One morning Katy's landlady found her on the floor of the back porch of the boarding house. She was unconscious and apparently had been there for several hours. An ambulance was called and Katy was taken to a hospital. A kind doctor who had taken care of her before knew that she needed financial help. He called the welfare department and told officials that Katy had made a fortune and lost it. She now was another name on the welfare rolls. After an examination, Katy was diagnosed as having had a stroke. Over a two-week period she began to show signs of improvement.

On March 5, 1947, Katy was transferred to Pineview Hospital. Her physical condition improved rapidly, but mentally she showed no signs of improvement. She was seventy-nine and now was living in the past.

Katy never forgot to say "please" when she asked for something and "thank you" when she received so much as a smile. Much of the time it was "please, dearie" and "thank you, dearie." She kept her hair neatly combed and never forgot a little rouge on her cheeks, but was much too extravagant with face powder.

I had been at Pineview only a few weeks when Katy called me over to her bed. With her eyes fairly dancing, she put her arm around my neck to pull me down and whisper in my ear: "Are you making any money, dearie?" I replied, "No, not much. This job is a lot of work and backaches, but the pay is not so much." Katy looked perplexed and was silent for several minutes before replying: "There is something wrong, dearie, because you do have beautiful girls here." I knew some of my nurses were pretty, but I was at a complete loss to know why that should affect their income. I gave Katy a loving pat on her cheek and left the room.

Several days later, when Katy was all made up for the day, she decided she would enjoy sitting in the big chair on the ladies' veranda. I helped her to the chair and adjusted the pillow behind her head. At the opposite end of the corridor was the men's veranda. An old man in his nineties came hobbling down the hall supported by canes, one in each hand. He found his chair. After getting himself in a position to sit, he took a long time to relax his stiff old body and get down. Finally, he sat with a resounding thud. Katy watched his every move. Her eyes grew larger and larger as she observed the old man taking his seat. Finally, she called out to me, "Come here, dearie!" Pointing her finger at the old man she said, "No wonder you aren't making any money."

That afternoon Katy had a visitor. He was a retired man from Anaconda, Montana, near Butte, and had known Katy during her days of prosperity. He brought her a box of candy and a basket of fruit. After his visit with Katy he had a long visit with me and told me the story of Katy's life. He left his telephone number with instructions that he was to be called if she ever needed anything. This man died soon after his visit to Pineview.

One of Missoula's women's organizations kept Katy supplied with powder, rouge, lipstick, hair pins, combs and costume jewelry, which she dearly loved. One afternoon a lady from Missoula who often called on the old folks stopped to visit Katy. Katy was neither in her bed nor in her chair on the veranda. The woman called me to help find her. We quietly pushed the door to the bathroom open and there was Katy, on her hands and knees, looking under the old-fashion bathtub. The tub, on legs, was about eight inches from the floor. Katy had a stick and was poking around under the tub. Tapping her on her bare rear and (her short gown opened in the back and separated as she bent over), I asked, "What on earth are you doing?" Katy was startled, but she rose to her feet and, in a soft, sweet voice, said, "You know, the governor spent the night with me last night and he slipped out and didn't tell me good-bye. I thought he might be hiding in here, the rascal." She hesitated and then added, "He will be wanting to come back and that is no way to treat a lady." The woman with me shook her head as she said, "Poor Katy, she just doesn't know what she is talking about, does she?" I replied, "No, she doesn't," but thought to myself, "Maybe she is just dreaming of yesteryear."

A roommate arrives

Miss Mary Copeland, a very small lady, was admitted to Pineview and given a bed in Katy's room. She was a welcome guest, for now Katy would have somebody to listen to her stories of her men friends and the many places she had visited on her world travels. Katy did not realize that Miss Copeland did not understand anything she told her. Miss Copeland only smiled and would nod her head occasionally.

Katy danced around Mary's bed like a butterfly. She even sang songs to her. Miss Copeland had no idea why her roommate was so friendly. Katy had her eyes on a number of Mary's belongings; she knew if she managed things just right, she would have them for herself.

When the supper trays were brought in, Katy volunteered to help Miss Copeland. Long ago Katy had lost her false teeth and had gone toothless. Now was her big chance. Mary had good-looking dentures and Katy offered to take them to the bathroom to clean them for her. Instead of putting them into the tooth mug after cleaning them, she put them into her own mouth. She went to the dresser and adjusted the mirror to get a good look at herself. They were loose, but if she held her mouth just right she could keep them in place.

The evening nurse entered the room, but Katy was so busy admiring herself and her new teeth she did not hear her. The nurse scarcely recognized Katy and finally noticed it was the teeth that made the difference. As soon as Katy was aware of the nurse's presence, she dove for her bed, jumped in and pulled the covers over her head.

The nurse left Katy alone and went to Miss Copeland's bed. Miss Copeland was doing an excellent job of gumming her baked potato. Her jaws were working at a terrific rate of speed. She seemed amused as she reached for another spoonful of her potato. She didn't utter a sound as she continued to eat. The nurse knew Katy would not come out of hiding to eat as long as she was in the room, so she quietly left. She returned in a half hour. Katy had eaten, but did not have the teeth in her mouth. A nurse spent the next hour hunting for Miss Copeland's teeth, but her search was to no avail. She posted a notice at the nurses' chart desk: *L O S T — Mary Copeland's Teeth.* Everybody was alerted to try to find them, but nobody did.

Three days later a doctor making his rounds and seeing patients approached Katy's bed. She had a smile for him. Her mouth was so full of teeth she could not talk. I didn't wish to create a disturbance so I slipped out of the room to find a nurse. I asked the nurse to find things to do in Katy's room, but not to let her out of her sight until the teeth were recovered and returned to the rightful owner.

Katy watched very carefully. When she thought the nurse was so busy with Miss Copeland that would not notice what she was doing, she slid out of bed like a cat and disappeared into the bathroom. The nurse tiptoed to the door, which was slightly ajar, and watched Katy carefully wrap the teeth in a wash cloth and place them far under the bath tub. The nurse quickly returned to Miss Copeland's bed and ignored Katy's activities until Katy was back in her own bed and had her face covered with the spread. The nurse went to the hiding place, got the teeth and returned them to Mary Copeland. Neither Mary nor the nurse ever mentioned the teeth, but our staff guarded them from then on.

Katy was a problem for the night nurses. She would get out of bed at all hours of the night and roam. Around two or three each morning the cookie jar in the nurses' dining room was a favorite destination.

Katy developed nephritis and began to fail rapidly. She was allergic to so many medicines that it was difficult to treat her. After several weeks of treatment for her kidney condition, her heart began to cause trouble. The last few days before her death, Katy slept most of the time. She never complained, always had a smile and whispered, "Yes, dearie, thank you, dearie."

I often thought as I looked from one patient to another and wondered which one I was going to be like when I was old, *I hope I shall be just like Katy. She is always happy and is always kind and courteous to everyone.*

Lester

Lester was admitted to Pineview Hospital on August 2, 1947. He was eighty-seven years of age and suffering from a long-standing heart ailment, among other things.

Lester and his wife had owned a large ranch in the Bitterroot Valley south of Missoula. They ran more than 1,200 head of white-faced cattle. The ranch produced ample hay to feed the cattle during winter months; Lester grazed them on federal domain during the summer for a small fee.

The couple had twin sons. They helped on the ranch during summers and went to school in Missoula during the winter. The boys graduated from Montana State University in time to enlist in the army during the First World War. Both were sent overseas. Neither returned. They were killed in action a few weeks apart.

The Depression of 1929 dealt another blow to these people. The price of cattle dropped drastically and each year Lester and his wife found themselves with fewer cattle and heavier debts. They sold their ranch in 1935; when all expenses were paid they had little left. They moved into town to find work. Lester worked as a carpenter for several years, making just enough money to support his wife and himself. In 1938 Lester was elected to serve as a county commissioner. He spent two days each week in that capacity and continued to do carpentering the rest of the time. His wife died in 1939 after a stroke.

Lester did an outstanding job as a public official. He had had problems and was very understanding of people and their troubles.

When he was brought to Pineview, he was an old man with a broken body and a broken spirit. He was put to bed and a doctor ordered "complete rest." That meant he must not get out of bed; it would be necessary for nurses to feed him. Lester was very cooperative and in a few weeks he could do everything for himself.

He responded to the love and care he received. He soon became somebody who gave a lot of moral support to other patients in his room, as well as to the people who worked at Pineview. Everyone called him "Dad" and he was proud of the title.

Lester had a wonderful bass voice and would sing by the hour. He joined the church groups that came on Sunday to sing for patients.

On March 16, 1950, at 2:30 in the afternoon, while "Dad" was taking his afternoon nap, he slipped away to join his wife and their two boys.

Louise

Louise was seventy-five years old when she came to Pineview. She weighed three-hundred-forty-two pounds and was a diabetic. She loved food more than anything.

Her husband had been dead for twelve years. She had a daughter, Anna, who was married and lived in Spokane, Washington. The daughter came twice a year to visit her mother, once in the spring and again in the fall.

Before coming to Pineview, and during one of Anna's spring visits, Louise put her affairs in order. She and Anna called on one of the morticians in Missoula and Louise made arrangements for her funeral and burial. She chose a casket but, because of her size, a special one had to be ordered. The original price quoted was $250, but when it was decided that an oversize casket would be needed, the price rose to $350.

Louise selected the shroud she thought was prettiest; it cost $19.95. She thought it was a real bargain. Flowers would be $25. (Louise was fond of flowers and the mortician promised her he would personally see that she had a large bouquet.)

The next item was the fee for the minister. Louise was told that would be strictly up to her. Without hesitation she said, "Put down ten dollars for him." She turned to Anna and whispered, "That's highway robbery, but I do want a good sermon." The mortician added, "I almost forgot. There is a five-dollar charge for someone to play the organ and sing." This met with Louise's approval.

The mortician added up the items, which came to a total of $409.95. Louise asked the mortician to turn his back while she got the money for him. She pulled up her long, full skirt, reached inside her stocking and pulled out a roll of bills. She carefully counted out $410, which she handed to the mortician. This time she turned her back as she slipped the remaining roll down inside her stocking. She complimented the mortician on knowing his business as she extended her hand for her five cents change. After a warm handshake, she departed with a feeling of satisfaction. She knew that things would be done right and just like she wanted.

Louise spent the next few days getting her little house rented. Anna packed all the things she wished to keep and sent them to Spokane. Louise gave the rest of her worldly possessions to friends and neighbors.

Louise was happy in her new home at Pineview. She grew fond of the employees and her fellow patients. She talked by the hour whether anyone listened or not. Anna's spring and fall visits were the highlights of her quiet life.

Louise had been at Pineview for three years when she began to fail. She lost her appetite and for weeks refused to eat. Only a small amount of food could be forced. Anna came to try to help the nurses care for her. She lost pound after pound and became very thin. She lived for almost a year with her body slowly wasting away. Pneumonia was the friend that finally took her away.

The mortician came to Pineview for Louise's body. He was surprised to find her below average in size. He didn't hide his amazement as he stared at the body.

At the funeral, I noticed that Louise had been placed in a standard-size casket. I never asked Anna if she was reimbursed the extra $100 for the specially ordered casket; Anna never mentioned it. Every other detail was as Louise had planned. The sermon was excellent, her shroud, music and flowers beautiful. Just as she wanted.

Aletha and Steve

Life never was monotonous at Pineview. There were surprises almost every day. One of the biggest jolts I experienced during my years at Pineview happened the morning that Aletha whispered in my ear that she was going to marry her friend, Steve.

Aletha was ninety-two, Steve eighty-nine. She had been married five times and had raised nineteen children. She told me she had had lots of experience and knew when real love was present. She also said, "After all these years and all the men I've courted, I surely must know when one of the opposite sex is in love with me. Steve is such a nice gentleman. My daughter tells me he has a brother who is wealthy and who has no family to leave his money to except Steve." She motioned for me to come closer; as she stopped her knitting she whispered, "The brother isn't so well of late."

Steve was married when he was a young man working as a buckaroo on a ranch in the Big Hole country. His wife was half Flathead Indian and half French. They went to the reservation near Arlee to see the Indians perform at a pow-wow. That was the first summer after their marriage.

The first night on the reservation, Steve's wife joined the Flatheads in their celebration. The last time he saw her was around midnight. She was dancing with a group of young people in a circle. They were holding hands, keeping step with the hum-drum music made by a dozen men beating on drums. They had danced for several hours without losing their enthusiasm. Steve sat on the ground where he could see his wife as she danced past him every few minutes. But she never looked his way. Steve became weary and dozed off for a moment. He suddenly became aware of his wife's absence and started to look for her. He questioned each dancer, but no one had seen her. Steve spent days hunting for his wife. He could not find anyone who knew anything about her whereabouts.

Each year at pow-wow time Steve returned to the reservation hoping he might find his wife. He never remarried, nor did he ever forget the beautiful girl who had shared with him the happiest months of his life.

So much of his time was spent looking for his wife that he never settled down to making and saving money for his old age. His brother, Bill, had worked hard, saved his money and had bought a sheep ranch in his younger days. He was two years older than Steve and had watched the years deal blows and heartaches to his younger brother. He devoted his years to raising sheep and selling them and wool. He never became involved with women.

Steve had always been independent and never accepted anything from his brother. He always said he wanted it that way so they would remain good friends.

It was the middle of May and sheep-shearers were busy on Bill's ranch. It was a pleasant day, so Bill thought he would help the boys. The exertion proved to be more than he could stand; he suffered a heart attack and died. He left his sheep ranch and his money to his brother.

June arrived at Pineview with more excitement than ever had been known. Aletha and Steve were married on a veranda of Pineview Hospital with all the employees and patients in attendance. A minister read from the Bible. As he said, "Steve and Aletha, I pronounce you man and wife," everything was still for a moment. Then the "celebration" broke loose.

The couple's possessions were packed into my car; after all the farewells were said, I drove the happy pair to their new home. They now had everything, including hired help to care for them. But most important of all, they had each other. I kissed them good-bye and agreed to come see them. I could not help wondering whether Steve took care of his marital status before marrying Aletha, but I decided that was not important.

Charley

C harley and his wife, Margaret, came to Missoula from Ohio. They bought twenty acres along the Clark Fork River. They worked hard and prospered. A son, Charles Jr., and a daughter, Mabel, were born soon after Charley and Margaret settled in Montana. Charley and Margaret were leaders in the Missoula community. They were active in the Methodist Church and took part in community affairs.

Charles Jr. and Mabel attended the state university after completing their high school in Missoula. Mabel was married the summer after she graduated. Charles studied journalism and moved to Seattle to work with his uncle on a newspaper. He was a thrifty and capable man. In time, he was part owner of one of Seattle's largest newspapers.

Charley and Margaret were successful over the years. They added more land to their original acreage. They started a dairy after selling their range cattle and buying Holstein milk cows. They soon had a herd of a hundred good-producing milkers.

One icy morning in 1937 as Margaret was returning home from grocery shopping in Missoula, her car skidded on ice. She was killed at a railroad crossing. Charley realized that the responsibility of operating the dairy was more than he could handle alone. He and Mabel did not get along very well and Mabel's husband never was accepted by Charley. Charley knew it would never be satisfactory to ask Mabel and her husband to become partners in his business.

A young couple from Canada moved to Missoula and learned that Charley needed help at the dairy. The Canadian man had considerable experience and Charley was happy to employ him as manager of the dairy.

Charley lived a very comfortable life. He had his living quarters in the front part of his house; the Canadian couple lived in back rooms, with two rooms upstairs.

During the winter of 1939-1940, Charley's health failed. He was finding it difficult to get around. He was becoming forgetful and confused at times. Mabel's husband suggested that he and his wife sell Charley's dairy and place the eighty-year-old man in a "home."

A man from Butte bought Charley's business in the late spring of 1940 for $63,000. Before Charley realized what was happening, he was out of business and was living in an old house near the Northern Pacific railroad with a woman who ran a boarding house for county indigents. Weeks passed before Charley knew that Mabel and her husband had his money and that the county was paying for his board. Charley was heart-broken; he prayed each day to die.

His rheumatism became worse each winter. With the passing of each year he became more helpless. The fall of 1948, he came to Pineview a fragile, helpless old man without money and without friends. When I asked him about relatives, he hesitated, dried the tears that had oozed from his faded and cloudy eyes, and replied, "No comment."

Mabel and her husband moved to Colorado, where they bought a ranch. They never returned to Missoula.

Charley liked the nurses at Pineview and appreciated all they did for him. He was bathed each morning. Baby oil was rubbed over each bony joint to prevent pressure sores. He would cry out with pain as he was carefully turned from side to side. He loved the kind night nurse, Della Packer, who turned him every hour all night long. He enjoyed visits from the cook, Pheroda Burnett. He would tell her in detail about all the good things she should make for him to eat. She would follow his orders to the letter, only to see his tray come back to the kitchen with only a few bites eaten.

"Grandpa" Charley's only pleasure was his pipeful of Prince Albert tobacco after his few bites of food. Often, when he had moments of feeling very

81

weak, he would ask for me and whisper his one special request: "I think it best that you look in my cupboard and bring me a wee bit of my wine." Each time he talked with me the conversation would end with another request: "And you promise you will sit with me and hold my hand while I die?" The answer was always, "Yes, Grandpa, I promise."

One early morning in January 1954, Grandpa called Della, the night nurse, and told her to call me. "Grandpa," the nurse said, "it's two o'clock in the morning; Marie is asleep." Charley said, "Do as I say. She promised me she would come when I sent for her. You had better hurry or I'll die before she gets here." Della obeyed. I was sitting at his bedside holding Grandpa's withered hand in less than twenty minutes. He peeked at me through half-closed eyes and said, "I knew you'd come — I believe tonight is the night. I feel very weak." I gave him a few drops of his wine. About three hours later, Charley opened his eyes wide and stared at me: "You can go back to bed now, I'm going to make it," he whispered. "Thank you for coming to me."

Two years passed. Each day, Grandpa grew more tired and weary. He sent for me once more. I sat at his bedside for hours whispering prayers in his ear. He slipped into eternity quietly, leaving Della and me on either side of his bed. We looked at each other, understanding what the other was thinking. Finally, I said, "It's not Mabel or Charles Jr. who will be missing this sweet old man. It's the nurses, the cooks, the laundry woman, the janitor, all my dedicated Pineview employees who have given him loving care all these years who will be missing him."

Mike

Mike was an eighty-year-old man who occupied one of the beds in a ward at Pineview. He had had a stroke that left him paralyzed on his left side.

He spent the last two years of his life at Pineview, but never was friendly with other patients. He talked very little to the employees. I tried several times to get a history to complete his record for the files. Each time he said the same thing: "No relatives, no friends, no religion." He gave his birthplace as a small town in Kentucky, but he could not remember the name. He refused to talk to any of the visiting clergymen. I had noticed that a man who operated a small business on the outskirts of Missoula had visited Mike at least twice during his two years at Pineview.

When Mike died, I notified the man. He came to Pineview to tell me that he wished to pay for Mike's funeral expenses. After all the business was taken care of, the man wanted to talk to me. He had never told anyone about Mike as long as Mike was alive. Now Mike was gone; the man wanted to share Mike's secret with someone who cared enough to listen.

Many years earlier, when Mike was a young man living in Chicago, he became involved with gangsters. He had been associated with them only a short time when he was ordered to kill a man. Mike had never done anything like that before; in his excitement, and with his inexperience, he killed the wrong man. He was terrified by his blunder, but was successful in finding the "right" victim. Mike proceeded to kill him.

On his way to meet his underworld boss to report his accomplishment, Mike saw a freight train coming down the tracks. He made a dash for it. He didn't care where the train was going. He realized the law would be after him, but, even worse than the law, the gang boss would be after him. He wanted to get as far away as possible. Mike didn't leave the empty boxcar until it reached Billings, Montana. He had decided to change his name and start life anew.

He was afraid to be seen, so he found a job on a ranch herding sheep. He spent his next forty years living the life of a hermit and tending sheep. He learned to love sheep. He began to suffer from rheumatism and found it increasingly difficult to walk the rocky hills with the sheep. He felt more secure with the passing of years and decided to live in town. He moved to Missoula and started to work as a handyman for the businessman who later came to see him at Pineview. Mike was a good worker and lived in a shack just behind the man's place of business.

One cold winter night when the temperature in Missoula dipped to well below zero, Mike's employer invited Mike to come into his house, where it was warmer. The men decided to have a drink of whiskey to help make the weather more tolerable. After several drinks Mike felt warm and cozy; a desire to talk overtook him. It was the first time in his life that he really felt like talking. He started at the beginning, with his joining with the gangsters, and never stopped until his entire story was complete. He even described his favorite sheep on the isolated range in eastern Montana. It was early morning when Mike finished; never once did he mention his family or his real name.

Mike's friend said good-bye to me and started out the door. He suddenly stopped and returned to my desk. He said in a low, quivering voice, "But, Marie, Mike was a good man." He turned and left, wiping tears from his cheeks.

Jane

Jane was born in New York City. She attended Columbia University and taught school for a number of years before marrying a dentist who practiced in New York.

They had been married for a number of years when they moved to Missoula. Jane's husband opened a practice. He loved the hunting and fishing that western Montana had to offer.

Jane taught Sunday school at a local church. She had no children and spent her time teaching the children of her church. Much of her time was devoted to taking care of homeless animals.

Jane's husband had a heart attack while elk hunting. He still was a young man. He died before rescuers could get him out of the mountains and into town. He left Jane with ample funds to take care of herself as long as she lived. At least the money would have lasted had Jane not been so generous in taking care of animals. She maintained a home for all homeless dogs and cats until her personal funds were exhausted. This happened to her before she realized her money had dwindled away.

Jane started teaching school for a living, but her health began to fail. After three years of teaching, she became ill in her classroom one morning. She was rushed to a hospital in Missoula. She had suffered a stroke and would be hospitalized for an extensive period.

Her beautiful home had to be sold to provide funds for her care. She had been ill for almost two years and her money was gone. Surprisingly, her friends were gone, also.

Jane was brought to Pineview to be cared for until there was room available for her in the Masonic Home in Helena. Months passed, and still there was no bed for her in Helena. Jane grew fond of everyone at Pineview and lost interest in going to Helena. She had learned to walk again; she loved to talk and visit with anyone who would take time to listen to her.

I noticed that Jane seemed depressed. I asked, "Jane, is something bothering you? Is there anything I can do for you?" The answer was yes. "I want to go to town so badly," she said. I told her I would take her next morning.

It was 10 o'clock when we got into my car and left for town.

"Jane, what do you want to buy that is so important?" I asked.

Jane would not say until we were downtown. She was like a child. Finally, she took my hand and held it for awhile. Then she whispered, "I have wanted a bottle of soda pop for so long, a bottle of orange crush. Marie, will you please, please get it for me?" I stopped at a store, went in and bought three bottles of orange soda. We sat in the car and watched people pass by as we sipped our sodas. Neither of us spoke a word; we just sat and watched people. An hour passed, then Jane said, "Marie, I love you more than anyone in this world. Let's go home."

Jane was tired, but happy. I put her to bed. As I was smoothing her pillow, I asked, "Jane, is there anything else I can do for you?" She replied, "Just let me kiss you for doing so much for me."

I left to check on other patients. I returned to Jane's room a few minutes later to tell her there was a bottle of orange crush in the icebox for her anytime she wanted it. I was shocked when I looked at Jane. I knew at once that she had quietly gone to be with her husband. As I lifted her hand, I said aloud, "Oh, thank God I took her to town for that soda. Her last wish was granted."

Tom

Tom made his home at Pineview for five years. He had been a successful businessman in Missoula for many years. He and his wife operated a laundry and dry-cleaning establishment. They had no children. They gave generously to their church, both in money and time. Tom was proud of a fifty-year pin that the Elks Lodge had presented him.

Tom and his wife owned a lovely home and thought their savings were ample to provide some comforts for their old age. Ten years of illness in their family changed things. Tom took his wife to specialists in different parts of the country. He was determined to find one who could restore health to the woman he loved so much. First, their savings were gone. Then the laundry and dry-cleaning business had to be sold. Finally, their home had to be sacrificed to provide funds to meet their obligations. Tom's wife had to stay in the hospital month after month with round-the-clock nurses to care for her.

T om was an old man and dispirited after the doctors, nurses and funeral bills were paid. He was broke. How could this happen? He had nothing now, except time, as he sat in a chair beside his bed at Pineview. He would say, "Yes, Marie, I'd do it all over again for her. She would have done the same for me. We always loved each other very much. No, I have no regrets." This seemed to be a comfort now. He knew he had done everything possible for his wife.

Months passed. Many of Tom's friends had died and the ones who were left did not have transportation, were not physically able, or found it too much of an effort, to come and visit Tom. A kind, elderly gentleman who made his home at Missoula's Elks Club was the only person left who called on Tom.

The man always brought Tom candy, chewing tobacco and rectal suppositories to aid in elimination.

As the years passed, Tom spent his days reminiscing about the laundry and his wife. He would "talk" to her, and also to their customers. He remembered them all. He seemed content as his mind wandered back to the happiest days of his life. He talked of his school days, playing ball, doing chores on the farm, his mother's home-made bread and her sugar cookies. He would ask why "women nowadays" couldn't cook like that.

He referred to me as "Mother" and called me frequently to help him with his problems: The broken shoe string, the suspender that had lost its stretch and no longer would hold up his trousers. He ceased asking his friend to bring candy, but he did want chewing tobacco. His requests for suppositories increased.

Tom did not sleep well. He would get out of bed to roam around at night. Della, the night nurse, would meet him in the building at all hours. He always was cooperative and would return to his room when requested to — if he was not pressured. He would become abusive and would fight if he was hurried in any way. Coping with him required endless patience.

For several days, Tom was extremely nervous and restless. He wanted "Mother" to do a hundred and one trivial things for him. He followed me around everywhere I went. Finally, I asked, "Tom, what on earth is wrong with you?" He sat down on a chair beside me and whispered, "Mother, you have to help me. I think I have cancer. There's a lump in my rectum that feels like a big potato. It's been growing bigger for days and my bowels won't move." He added, "You know, Mother, I always have trouble with my bowels. Those suppositories used to do me good, but not anymore. I feel awful, Mother. Do something for me, please."

I took Tom to his room and helped him undress. He was like a child. I remembered attending a lecture given by a specialist in geriatrics. He told the class that one of the signs of approaching old age was the great concern over one's bowels. If a patient's bowels moved once a day, they were suffering from constipation. If they moved twice a day, they were ready to die from diarrhea.

Poor Tom was really having bowel trouble and I felt I must help him. I told him I would insert one of his suppositories for him and examine his rectum for that "potato." I stood beside his bed talking to him as I unwrapped the tinfoil from the suppository. He was watching my every move, his eyes getting bigger and bigger. As I completed the procedure, Tom found enough voice to exclaim, "Mother, are you supposed to take that silver stuff off?"

The examination revealed a round ball of packed foil as large as a golf ball. I called one of the nurses to show her the shining silver "potato" that Tom thought was cancer. I asked the nurse to take plenty of time in removing this foreign body from Tom's rectum so as not to cause any more distress than necessary. I also asked that Tom's friend be instructed to deliver the suppositories to the nurse on duty so she could see that they were properly administered. Tom's condition improved at once; he had no more trouble with that particular ailment.

He continued to roam through the hospital and talk to his imaginary friends. He was very dependent on the nurses and they were extremely kind and patient with him.

Tom had a heart attack one night just before Easter. The doctor came and I was called to sit at Tom's bedside as I had promised him many times I would do. Tom was not alone when he left this world. The entire staff was in his room to say good-bye. Tears were in the eyes of everyone.

Tom was buried beside his wife under a tall pine tree in the Missoula cemetery.

Another Tom

This Tom was born in Altoona, Pennsylvania. His father, like other men in the town, worked hard in the coal mines. He expected his two sons to work just as hard.

Tom had gone to school and finished the third grade when his father insisted he was old enough to go to work. He thought Tom had had enough schooling and that Tom was such a big boy he should be doing manual labor. When Tom was twelve he went to work for a blacksmith. He brought his paycheck home each payday and handed it over to his father.

At age fourteen, Tom decided to leave home. One night after his father, mother and younger brother had gone to sleep, he slipped out of bed. He placed a note that he had written the day before on the kitchen table, then cautiously opened the kitchen door and disappeared into the darkness. He threw back his shoulders and breathed deeply of the cool air as he thought, *Now I am a man.* He stopped for a moment and stared back toward the house. *Good-bye, Ma and Joe,* he thought. *To hell with you, Pa.* Then he was gone.

When his mother went to the kitchen to prepare breakfast for her husband and sons, she saw the folded white paper at her husband's place at the table. She unfolded it and read:

> **Dear Pa and Ma and Joe,**
> **I am leaving home tonight for a far-away land to seek my fortune. You won't see me again until I have found it. I'll come home then.**
>
> **Your son,**
> **Tom**

Tears streamed down the mother's cheeks as she cooked the eggs. She begged her husband to try and find Tom and bring him home. He only laughed and said, "That boy will come home when he gets hungry." He was mistaken. Tom did not return.

Tom was big for his age and readily made friends with men on the freight trains. There were many hoboes on the freights and in the hobo camps along the railroads. Tom traveled in this fashion from Altoona to Omaha, Nebraska. He decided he would stop there and find work to make enough money to buy food on the rest of his journey.

The hobo method of travel was to eat while in one of the camps. But, while traveling, there was no food. Tom did not like that. He needed food daily to satisfy his growing body.

He found a job shoveling coal from freight cars into wagons. He worked several weeks at the job and ate well at a cafe next to the station.

His next trip was from Omaha to Cheyenne, Wyoming. He again left the freight train and found a job for the winter feeding sheep on a large ranch just north of Cheyenne. When spring came, Tom was ready to travel again. From Cheyenne he went to Ogden, Utah. He met a fellow traveler on that trip, a man who had worked in the copper mines in Butte, Montana, and was on his way back to them. Tom decided to go with him.

After twenty years of working hard and living high, Tom and his friend moved on to Montana's Bitterroot mountain range and started to work in the timber. They snaked big logs down the mountainside and helped load them onto wagons that took them into Stevensville, Montana, to a lumber mill. This was extremely hard work, but they were fed well. Also, the timberjacks were a happy-go-lucky bunch that enjoyed that kind of life.

The men worked in the mountains all summer and came to town to spend the winter. They all lived at a boarding house. The woman who owned it was a good cook, kept her place plenty warm, and allowed them to drink all the whiskey they wanted as long as they kept their bills paid.

One Saturday night Tom got so drunk that he lost control of himself. As a rule he could drink a great deal, but he always was a gentleman. This night, though, he began to pick men up and toss them around. He had his fun doing that, then started getting rough with the women. When he picked up the boarding house owner and held her high in the air with her head touching the ceiling, she thought it was time to do something. She called the sheriff and told him to take Tom away for the rest of the night. The sheriff knew he could not take Tom by force; after talking to him for some time, the sheriff took Tom to jail.

The jail was a small, square, log cabin with one tiny window. There was no bed or furniture of any kind, only a wooden box used for a chair. Tom still had a surplus of energy and could not sit still. He put his shoulder against the wall and pushed with all his might. He felt the little log house loosening from its foundation, so he kept heaving until he pushed it over.

It was only a few feet to the Bitterroot River. Tom kept the jailhouse "rolling" until he heard what he called "a heck of a splash." Down the river went the Stevensville jail. It was too dark for Tom to see it, but he could hear logs breaking away from each other. He knew the jail soon would be in a hundred pieces. He found his way back to his seat on the wooden box.

At sunrise the sheriff walked down to his prisoner's quarters. What a surprise he got to see Tom sitting there on the wooden box out in the open! He was sure the jailhouse was there, but after rubbing his eyes almost out of his head he knew Tom had pushed it into the river. Now Tom was sitting in front of him singing "Sweet Adeline." The sheriff knew Tom was as strong as a bull, but he never dreamed Tom could cheat future prisoners out of a home in such a short time.

Tom spent the rest of his working years in the Bitterroot mountains. He worked summers and spent the long, cold winters in Stevensville at the boarding house. He made money during the summer and spent every dime of it during the winter.

He was admitted to Pineview Hospital with acute nephritis. After one of Tom's severe attacks of hard chills and fever, I was telling a doctor some of the stories Tom had told me. After I finished, the doctor laughed and said, "You know, I've known him for years." It was the doctor's turn to tell a story about Tom.

It was a warm Saturday night in July and all the timberjacks had come to town for the weekend. The doctor had been called from Missoula to Stevensville on a baby case. It was understood that the doctor could always have the bed in a particular corner of the big sleeping room anytime he wanted to stay all night at the boarding house. He had unhitched his horses from his buggy, had put them in the barn and had gone to bed. He was tired after a difficult delivery and was going to sleep until morning. He would check on the mother and newborn baby before returning to Missoula.

The doctor had gone to sleep, but was awakened by a half-dozen timberjacks coming up to bed. Everything was quiet for a while, then the doctor heard Tom say, "Damn it to hell!" as Tom's feet hit the floor. Tom made a dash for the window and raised it to the top with a bang. He hung his head out and, with a long, loud regurgitating noise, started to vomit. Below his window was an alfalfa field full of pigs. After each loud regurgitation, the pigs would squeal as they fought over the food that was landing on the ground below the window. This went on and on; the more Tom would vomit, the more the pigs would squeal. Finally, Tom raised his head and yelled, "Quit your fighting, you sons-a-bitches, there'll be plenty for all!" With that he emptied his stomach of the last of its contents.

He closed the window and found his way back to bed. As he was pulling the blanket over him he said, "Pardon me, doctor, that damn cheap liquor made me sick."

When Tom told me his life story, I asked him if he had ever gone back to Altoona. He looked up at me and with a big laugh said, "I'll go back to see my ma and pa and Joe when I find my fortune. You know that, don't you?" He was eighty-eight years old and never had heard a word from his folks. Nor had they heard from him.

Tom passed away quietly one Sunday morning holding my hand. His last words were, "I hate to leave my buddies here, you've all been so damn good to me." The employees at Pineview contributed to Tom's funeral. He had a dark gray suit and a new white shirt with a dark red tie. His white hair, so neatly combed, gave him the appearance of a real aristocrat.

A kind woman from Missoula, and a good friend of all the old folks, played beautiful organ music. The minister talked about "Life beyond this earth." He talked to the ten hospital employees as though he were talking to hundreds of mourners.

I stood and bid farewell to a patient who always had been a perfect gentleman to all the personnel at the hospital. I knew he had recognized our resident, Katherine, as Madam Katherine from Butte when he saw her at Pineview. But, yes, he was a gentleman.

Harry

I interviewed Harry, sixty-seven, a pale, thin man with swollen, deformed hands and feet, a few days after I took over the operation at Pineview Hospital. Very little information was obtained at the time of admission. Harry was a sullen person and did not think it anyone's business concerning his private life. He was in too much pain to be bothered with foolish questions. However, he did volunteer the information that he had come West from the East to work in the mountains.

He would work hard when weather permitted. He saved his money until snow forced the logging camps to close, then he would move to town to spend the winter. Several timberjacks and Harry would live in a cheap boarding house, where they drank and played poker until spring. As soon as roads were passable, they returned to the mountains. This was routine year in and year out for twenty years of Harry's life. He enjoyed every day of it.

He grew older and his joints became stiff and sore. He found it difficult to walk and he knew he would not be able to return to the mountains for another season of hard work. The pain was so severe he had to seek medical attention. He applied for assistance and was referred to a doctor. After several weeks of treatment with little or no improvement, Harry was admitted to Pineview Hospital for care.

His condition grew worse and he was unable to get out of bed without help. He found it too much of a burden to feed himself because of the pain and increased deformity in his hands. Harry always was very quiet and did not encourage conversation with the other three patients in his ward or with the employees who took care of him. The nurses tried to cheer him with funny little happenings of the hospital, but he did not show interest.

His fellow roommates enjoyed watching sporting events on television, but Harry would pull the covers over his face. The cook would visit him and try to interest him in food. He ate very little and would not eat anything that was not spoon-fed to him. Ice cream was his favorite food and he thrived on it.

Harry enjoyed music and would ask a man who visited from town to play a few of his favorite numbers. When the man learned that his music meant so much to Harry, he would make an extra trip each week to play for him. He never missed playing "Red

River Valley" and "Take Me Home Again Kathleen."
I noticed tears on Harry's cheeks when these numbers
were played. I often wondered why these songs
caused him to be so emotional. Harry was growing
more helpless and weaker each week. His only
interest was the piano player's visits. He would ask
each day, "Will he be here tonight to play for me?"

The night nurse reported that Harry had had a
restless night. His temperature was slightly
elevated and he was listless. He ate very little
(less than usual) breakfast and complained of a dull
pain in his chest. The doctor was notified of the
change in Harry's condition and he came at once to
check him. He found a slightly congested area in the
lower left chest. The medication ordered by the doctor
was started and Harry seemed to be more comfortable.

I spent most of the next two days at Harry's
bedside. The third day he seemed much weaker and
his mind would wander back to the lumber camps in
the mountains. On several occasions he called for
"Harry." He referred to me as "Ella."

The doctor examined Harry again and his
condition was listed as serious. I remembered a small,
badly worn valise in the bottom drawer of Harry's
bedside table. He would never let anyone touch it. I
decided to slip this little satchel out to my office and
examine its contents as soon as Harry went to sleep. If
there were any relatives, they certainly should be
notified as to his condition. I knew Harry had not
mailed or received a letter during the time he had been
in the hospital. But why should he be calling for

99

"Harry" in his delirium and why should he call me "Ella?" He had insisted over and over that there were no known relatives.

It was noon before I tip-toed out of the ward with the old valise. I sat down at my desk and, after tugging at the rusty lock, it came open. I found several empty snoose cans, a bunch of rusty keys and a half-dozen soiled, red bandana handkerchiefs. In an empty can I found an old envelope addressed to Harry Conway Jr., 1411 Elm Street, Buffalo, New York. Inside the envelope was a yellow sheet of paper. The writing on it was in pencil and so dim with age it could not be read. After close examination, I saw that the only information distinguishable was the date, September 3, 1927. The place was Huron, Montana, Saw Mill #2. The message began, **"My dear son Harry, for a long time I have . . ."** There it ended. The rest of the sheet of paper was blank from soil and discoloration.

I went to the telephone and placed a person-to-person call to Harry Conway Jr. at 1411 Elm Street, Buffalo, New York. I was never more surprised than when the operator said, "I have him on the line." I explained all the details concerning my patient to the man at the other end of the line. I could tell that the man I was talking to was most upset and at a complete loss for words. He could not talk coherently and I was as confused as he seemed to be. Finally, I asked him if he knew anyone by the name of "Ella." He replied, "Oh, yes, that is my Aunt Ella Stricker, my father's sister. She lives in Pittsburgh." The man asked me if

100

he might call me back in a short while. He needed to collect his wits. I knew this man was in a state of shock and told him I would stand by for his call.

Less than an hour had passed when a call came from Ella Stricker in Pittsburgh. She was so excited she could hardly talk. She explained to me that she was sure this man at Pineview was her brother. This is the story she told:

Twenty-two years earlier, Harry Conway Sr. ate his breakfast with his wife, took his lunch pail and said, "Good-bye." He had done this daily for many years. He worked in the coal mines in Pennsylvania to support his wife and thirteen children. Harry Conway did not report for work, nor did he come home to his wife and children that night.

The search for him went on for weeks and months. After a year had passed and no trace of him had been found, he was officially declared dead. His family and friends accepted this with the exception of his son, Harry Jr., and his sister, Ella. They insisted that some day he would come home.

The children grew up, married and established their own homes. His wife moved to South Carolina to be near one of her daughters. Mrs. Stricker said she would come at once if her brother wanted her. She felt that Harry Jr. would come to be with his father, too. She added that she would talk to her nephew again and would call me and tell me of their decision. She also asked me to talk with her brother and find out if he wanted them to come. She wanted me to tell Harry that she loved him very much and wanted to be with him to help take care of him.

I sat by Harry's bedside and pleaded with him to say something that I could tell his family when they called again. He was sullen and would not answer. I told him over and over that his son wanted to see him and talk to him. The clock on the wall ticked away the minutes. They seemed like hours. I could hardly hear the telephone in my office ringing when Harry, with tears streaming down his face, grabbed me by the hand and said, "Please, tell my son I want to see him just as much as he wants to see me. Tell him I have so much to tell him and that I have always known that he and Ella would understand."

That was a happy moment for me. I at least had a message from the father of this man who was far away. It would mean so much to him. I repeated very carefully to him each word his father had said. He did not try to hide his grief or his happiness. He wept aloud as he said, "Oh, God, thank you, thank you." He added, "All these years I've prayed that some day I would find my father. And now my prayers have been answered." I could not control my tears as I listened to this man on the telephone line who was more than two-thousand miles away. He told me that he and his aunt would leave Pittsburgh the next morning to come to his father's bedside; when Harry was able to travel, they would take him home.

I returned to Harry with the good news. Harry's tired old face was radiant with happiness. He was pleased that they wanted to take him home.

102

Harry talked freely of his days in Pennsylvania with his family and of his working in the coal mines. He talked for almost an hour. Then, taking my hand, he thanked me for the things the nurses and I had done for him. He said he was tired and wanted to go to sleep, but would like to see the minister first.

The minister was pleased when I called him. He talked with Harry for some time and was elated to find his attitude changed. They prayed together, then the minister left. I returned to Harry's bedside to find his sullen expression gone. It had been replaced with smiles of peace and contentment.

I sat by Harry's bed while he slept. I was almost asleep, myself, when Harry suddenly reached for my hand. He had a gray pallor over his face as his head sank deeper into the pillow. His eyes looked straight into my face as he said with a smile, "I'm going home, I'm going home." A few shallow gasps and Harry slipped into eternity.

I did not know where I was going to get the courage to call Harry's son and tell him that his father was gone. I closed my eyes as I held Harry's motionless hand and asked God to give me strength to carry on my duties and to help me choose the right words to say to Harry's son.

The next morning I went to the mortuary to make arrangements to send Harry home to Pennsylvania. I selected the casket and a dark blue suit. Underwear and socks were needed. The mortician asked me to bring any clothing that Harry might have had. I didn't tell him that Harry had nothing fit for use.

I went to the Missoula Mercantile to make the necessary purchases; I would pay for the things and say nothing. I asked the salesman for a suit of long underwear and a pair of dark socks. He spent much time explaining to me about the bargain of buying two suits of underwear. He could not understand why I was not interested in the economy of his suggestion. He wrapped the one suit with the socks and I returned to the mortuary.

Harry's friend, the piano player, left work early that day and met the minister and the nurses from Pineview at the mortuary. The minister had a beautiful service and the piano player never did a better job with "Red River Valley."

The minister was back at his church, the piano player had gone home and the nurses had returned to Pineview as I stood alone on the platform of the railroad station and watched as the wooden box was carefully placed in the baggage car. As it disappeared through the car's doorway, I raised my hand to wave good-bye to my patient, who had for so long been surrounded by mystery. Now, after time had run out, he was going back home to Pennsylvania to a heartbroken son and sister. I could not help wondering why this man had left home, his wife and his thirteen children to lose himself among tall pines. There must have been a reason.

The train slowly moved along the track for a few yards, then gained speed as it rounded a bend two miles away. A feeling of utter panic filled me when all I could see was the red light on the back of the observation car. I asked myself, "Is this the right man I'm sending—to the right son? Will he come back C.O.D.?"

I did not sleep that night. I spent most of the night "on the train" with Harry and the balance with the son and the sister. As the sun started to rise next morning, I decided the man in the casket just had to be the right man. I fell asleep a few minutes before having to get up to start another day.

Five days later I received an air-mail letter from Harry Conway Jr. He was thanking me and the staff of Pineview for all that had been done for his father. I looked heavenward and whispered, "Thank you, dear God."

"I always wanted to be a nurse; it was a lifelong ambition."

—Marie McNeilly

Appendix

The poor farm cemetery

Two students, Shawn Moran and Amy Harper, once spoke with a man named Charles Keim (not Charles J. Keim, the writer) about his memories of the Missoula County Poor Farm.

Mr. Keim was about thirteen at the time his father, F.M. Keim, was poor farm superintendent. Charles Keim lived with his family at the farm during the winter of 1917-18. He could not remember ever seeing women or children there; most residents were Caucasian males and a small number of Chinese.

Mr. Keim remembered four or five Chinese burials taking place when he was at the farm. Bodies were taken to the cemetery in a horse-drawn wagon. Wooden caskets were supplied by the Marsh and Powell Funeral Home. Graves had no markers except for an occasional wooden cross. The Chinese would have a barbecue on top of the new graves.

Mr. Keim said that instead of decorating grave sites with flowers, as is the European custom, the Chinese placed scarves, ornamental trinkets, coins, and even food on the graves. Mr. Keim remembered only one cemetery. He believed the Chinese may have been buried in a separate corner of the cemetery, but he did not think they had a separate cemetery.

Burials at the poor farm cemetery
By Patrick Rennie & Thomas Estenson

We undertook this research in an attempt to identify the human skeletal remains disinterred in the summer of 1989 from Potters Field, a cemetery on the former grounds of the Missoula County Poor Farm, pest house and detention hospital.

Unfortunately, documentation regarding a significant number of burials either was not made at the time of interment or has not been preserved. The records that exist give little information pertinent to identification. Because of this, we determined that no identification could be made that would be more than wholly speculative.

In this section, we will present information obtained from historical records. It consists of five parts: Number of Burials, Race, Sex, Age and Cause of Death. Because of the dearth of records, any conclusions will be tentative and fairly subjective. The data presented came from the following sources:

Coroner's Record (prior to 1896)
Coroner's Report, 1896-1908
Coroner's Report, 1911-1920
Coroner's Report, 1921-1932
Auditor's Poor House Records, 1891-1896
Poor Farm Record, 1923-1926
County Farm Record, 1929-1932
Detention Hospital Records, 1927-1931
Missoula County Hospital Register, 1930-1931
Livingston, Malletta & Geraghty Funeral Home Records, 1901-1933

We obtained additional information from county commissioners' records, the *Missoulian* and U.S. Census reports.

Number of Burials

The four coroner's reports, and records from the Livingston, Malletta & Geraghty Funeral Home, contain the most accurate indications of burials at Potters Field. In the coroner's reports, there generally is some notation under the heading "Disposition of Body" that indicates the remains were sent to relatives, turned over to a local mortician or "Buried County Poor Farm." (Those instances in which this heading was left blank are not considered in the figures presented here, although it is possible that some of these may represent burials at Potters Field.) Coroner's reports usually were only filed in cases of accidents, suspicious deaths or found bodies.

No deaths occurring in hospitals under other circumstances, or otherwise considered "natural," were noted. In particular, no reports were filed regarding deaths at the county institutions. We tried to cross-reference known deaths at the poor farm with no success. The coroner's reports definitely list the following number of burials at Potters Field:

Record A (prior to 1896) 2
Coroner's report, 1896-1908 40
(1909-1910, no record)
Coroner's report, 1911-1920.................. 90
Coroner's report, 1921-1932 7
                                                    Total 139

The last notation from the coroner's reports indicating burial at Potter's Field is dated June 6, 1923.

Information in the coroner's reports is supplemented by records from Livingston, Malletta & Geraghty. The funeral home records list individuals who died in area hospitals or under natural circumstances. They have no records prior to 1901; their few records for the periods 1901 through 1906, and after 1919, would indicate that other mortuaries may have been handling the majority of Potters Field burials during those times. The Livingston, Malletta & Geraghty records indicate the following number of burials (mostly coincident with the coroner's reports):

1901 4	1912 16	1923 3
1902 1	1913 22	1924 4
1903 1	1914 26	1925 7
1904 12	1915 18	1926 4
1905 9	1916 31	1927 5
1906 7	1917 32	1928 3
1907 32	1918 38	1929 0
1908 63	1919 15	1930 1
1909 37	1920 3	1931 1
1910 18	1921 10	1932 0
1911 34	1922 8	1933 3

The significant number of deaths in 1908 resulted from a typhoid epidemic; those during the 1916-1918 period were from influenza.

Little documentation exists from the county poor farm. The records that do exist list 13 deaths during 1891-96, 5 during 1923-26, and 4 during 1929-32. However, this sample may not accurately reflect the total, since names disappear from the registry without notation, or individuals are shown as being transferred to the county hospital or to St. Patrick Hospital with no further history.

Since the population of the poor farm generally was elderly—the average age from the register of March 1917 was 63; from August 1928 it was 71—the mortality rate was probably high. Absence of documentation makes an exact count impossible.

The County Hospital Registry for 1930-1931 lists 27 deaths, with one specific notation, on January 23, 1930, that burial was to be on the county farm. No extrapolation for the other deaths can be made from this single notation, although it is indicative that at least some deceased patients were being buried at Potters Field. The detention hospital records from 1927-31 list two deaths but give no disposition of the remains.

One further fact should be noted: The poor farm was almost exclusively a male residence; the county made provisions to support females in other environments. However, at death, women under county care often were buried in Potters Field.

In summary, no exact determination of the number of burials can be made from county records. The extant records document 487 burials. However, the records prior to 1907 and after 1919 lack detail. Further, it is not clear that the data from 1907 through 1919 are inclusive. A conservative estimate to account for the missing information would increase the number of burials by 20 percent, to around 600. A more subjective estimate would increase the number by 50 percent to about 750 burials.

Race

No determination of race can be made from any of the historical records other than coroner's reports and funeral home records. Descriptions in those reports, other than name (when known) and age, are absent except under unusual circumstances. Apparently race, when other than white, qualified as an unusual circumstance since it was noted in 19 entries. Of the 139 individuals in the records, 3 are listed as Indian, 4 as Negro, and 12 as Chinese. (Chinese ceased to be buried in Potter's Field after 1908 per the commissioner's report of April 6, 1908, although they apparently continued to be buried elsewhere on the county's grounds. These numbers are consistent with the county's demographics. The U.S. Census report of 1910 for Missoula County lists 22,032 residents. Of this number, 133 are listed as "Negro" and 1,431 are listed under a single category of "Chinese, Japanese and Indian."

Sex
Only 21 adult females were listed in the historic records, perhaps a concomitant of the types of deaths investigated. This obviously is not representative of the demographics. The 1910 census shows 14,640 males and 8,956 females in Missoula County. Undoubtedly, some females were part of the unknown burials, although probably in a similarly smaller percentage than their composition of the overall population, since they were less likely to be transients and more likely to have had relatives or church affiliations that would have seen to their burials. It is doubtful that more than 10 percent of

the burials were female, with 5 percent a more likely figure.

Age
The records include 16 infants with no sex listed, seven females and sixteen males up to 9 years of age, and one female and two males from the age of 10 to 19. The rest of the burials that took place at Potters Field were for adults.

Ages are indicated for 350 individuals, with a mean of 48 years. (Where estimates were listed, an average of the range was used: 40 were 20 to 29; 81 were 30 to 39; 71 were 40 to 49; 59 were 50 to 59; 42 were 60 to 69, and 31 were over 70.) Unrecorded deaths from county institutions would have been significantly older. The poor house record from 1891-1896 has ages listed for 12 residents who died, at an average age of 54. As noted above, the average age of residents in 1917 was 63; in 1928 it was 71. It is, of course, not unexpected to have an elderly population represented in a cemetery.

Cause of Death
The unknown burials from the county institutions are presumed to be due to disease and old age. The known data from their records:

Auditor's Pest House Record, 1891-1896
1 paralysis
1 dropsy
1 asthma

1 hit by train
1 old age
1 Bright's disease
1 consumption
1 disability
1 liver disease
4 no entry

Poor Farm Record, 1923-1926
5 no entry

County Farm Record, 1929-1932
1 crippled
1 blind
2 senile

Detention Hospital Records, 1927-1931
2 syphilis

*Missoula County Hospital Register, 1930-
1931*
1 scarlet fever
26 no entry

*Summary of the causes of death from
coroner's reports and records of the Livingston,
Malletta & Geraghty Funeral Home:*
Hit by trains (other than suicide) 56
Listed as intoxicated 12
Suicide 25
Poison 8
Firearms 4

Knife 4
Hanging 2
Auto 1
No entry.. 2
Drowning 26
Listed as intoxicated 3
Alcoholism... 22
Natural causes 10
Accidents 6
Firearms 6
Burned.. 4
Beaten 3
Disease 3
Exposure 5
Excessive use of morphine 2
Hanging 2
Pneumonia 29
Typhoid... 20
Tuberculosis 15
Cancer.. 11
Myocarditis 10
Consumption 8
Hemorrhage 8
Nephritis 7
Apoplexy 5
Trees falling 3
Diphtheria 3
Auto accident 3
Rheumatism 3
Influenza... 3
Meningitis 3
Septicemia 2

Heart failure 2
Skull fracture 3
Arteriosclerosis 2
Bright's disease 2
Peritonitis 2
Abscess of brain 1
Measles 1
Brain concussion 2
Morphine poisoning 1
Blood poisoning 2
Hit by a rock 1
Broken neck 1
Infection 1
Abscess 1
Pulmonary edema 1
Tumor 1
Dilation of heart 1
Diabetes 1
Malignant edema 1
Gangrene 1
Exhaustion 1
Aneurism 1
Ulcer 1
Respiratory paralysis 1
Heat exhaustion 1
Liver trouble 1
Dropsy 1
Stopping of breath 1
Shock 1
Cocaine poisoning 1
Small pox 1
Spotted fever 1

During childbirth 1

The Western Montana Dairy Breeders Association
By Don Wold

The Western Montana Dairy Breeders Association was a farmers' cooperative formed in 1947. At that time there were many small dairy farmers in western Montana; there also was a need to improve the quality of dairy cattle so that higher milk production could be attained. The Orchard Homes and Target Range areas of Missoula consisted mainly of five- and ten-acre tracts; families living on these tracts each had a couple of dairy cows.

It was not economical for farmers with small numbers of dairy cattle to purchase a quality bull to upgrade their herds. So, the farmers banded together; with the help of the

118

Montana State Extension Service and Montana State University, they formed an artifical breeding cooperative. Oscar Tretsven from the state university and A.R. "Tony" Rollin of the extension service worked with the farmers in forming the cooperative, the Western Montana Dairy Breeders Association.

Since Missoula was the hub of the five valleys, it was logical to headquarter the cooperative in Missoula.

At that time, the county poor farm was located up the east Rattlesnake on 40 acres. The land was not in use. Through the efforts of Rollin and some local dairymen, the county commissioners were persuaded to turn the ground over to the new cooperative on a lease basis.

To finance the operation, both common and preferred stock were sold. Each member who joined the cooperative paid $10 for a share of common stock and was entitled to one vote. The creameries of western Montana generously purchased preferred stock at $100 per share to help the venture get off the ground.

The board of directors included one member from Missoula County, two from Ravalli County, two from Lake County and one from Flathead County. A prominent dairyman from Ravalli County, Paul Spannuth, was elected president of the association. Paul had a very keen mind and devoted much time to the organization.

Under the supervision of Oscar Tretsven, facilities were constructed to house the bulls and a laboratory was set up. Ten bulls were purchased — Holstein, Guernsey and Jersey breeds.

A crew was hired to care for the animals and manage the operation. Two inseminators were hired for both Ravalli and Lake counties, and one each for Missoula and Flathead counties. Semen was collected and processed at the bull farm every other morning. It was diluted with skim milk, poured into glass vials, and placed in pint Thermos bottles containing ice. The Thermos bottles were packed in insulated cardboard boxes and shipped by bus to the various inseminators.

From time to time the bull ring was upgraded with a young bull with a proven background. The aim of the association was to provide its members with the best affordable bloodlines available.

During the late 1940s and early 1950s, dairy cow numbers in western Montana dropped dramatically. The small dairymen went out of business and the milk-producing business went into the hands of large operators. For these reasons, it was not economical for the Western Montana Dairy Breeders Association to operate. Its existence ceased in 1953.

*"As long as I am here,
there will be no more going
to sleep hungry."*

—Marie McNeilly

"People from different cultures lived on 'The Poor Farm' located here from 1888-1930. After their deaths they were buried, but over the years their grave markers have disappeared. The indentations that cover this land are evidence of the grave sites. Through this memorial we hope you will remember the individual man, woman and child; the poor, the forgotten."

—Inscription at Rattlesnake School Graveyard Memorial, Missoula, Montana